T
BUTT &
THIGHS
WORKOUT
BOOK

THE LITTLE
BUTT &
THIGHS
WORKOUT
BOOK

ERIKA DILLMAN

WARNER BOOKS

NEW YORK   BOSTON

Neither these exercises and programs nor any other exercise program should be followed without first consulting a health care professional. If you have any special conditions requiring attention, you should consult with your health care professional regularly regarding possible modification of the program contained in this book.

The Little Butt & Thighs Workout Book™ is part of the "Little Book" series owned by Warner Books. All rights to the series and the trade dress are the property of Warner Books, Inc.

Warner Books

Time Warner Book Group
1271 Avenue of the Americas, New York, NY 10020
Visit our Web site at www.twbookmark.com

Printed in the United States of America

First Edition: March 2005

10 9 8 7 6 5 4 3 2 1

Library of Congress Cataloging-in-Publication Data
Dillman, Erika.
        The little butt & thighs workout book / Erika Dillman.—1st ed.
            p. cm.
        Summary: "A concise approach to toning two of the most stubborn areas of the body"—Provided by publisher.
        Includes bibliographical references.
        ISBN 0-446-67998-4
    1. Buttocks exercises. 2. Leg exercises. I. Title.
        GV508.D553 2005
        613.7'1888—dc22

                                                                    2004023549

Book design and text composition by L&G McRee
Cover design by Rachel McClain
Text illustrations by Emma Vokurka

Acknowledgments

Thanks to the following people for their contributions to *The Little Butt & Thighs Workout Book*:

My agent, Anne Depue, my editor, Diana Baroni, assistant editor Leila Porteous, and my friends and family for their continued support.

Emma Vokurka for her wonderful illustrations.

Debby Heath and Stephanie Molliconi for test-driving all of the exercises. Ted Johnson, Susan Huney, and Jill Irwin for their feedback on early drafts.

And special thanks to all the health and fitness experts who shared their time, knowledge, and expertise with me during the research and writing of this book. Their input has been invalu-

ACKNOWLEDGMENTS

able: Darcy Norman, licensed physical therapist, certified athletic trainer, and certified strength and conditioning specialist (CSCS) at Athletes' Performance; Michael Porter, M.S., ACSM-certified health and fitness instructor and certified strength and conditioning specialist (CSCS); Aaron Branam, ACSM-certified personal trainer and health and fitness instructor, certified strength and conditioning specialist (CSCS), and director of fitness operations at Seattle Athletic Club; Wayne Westcott, Ph.D., author and fitness research director at the South Shore YMCA in Quincy, Massachusetts; Amanda Gwinnup Carlson, M.S., R.D., and performance nutrition manager and research coordinator at Athletes' Performance.

Contents

CONTENTS

THE LITTLE
BUTT &
THIGHS
WORKOUT
BOOK

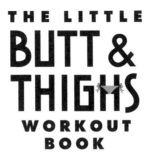

Welcome to *The Little Butt & Thighs Workout Book*

Firm Up, Shape Up

Does my butt look big in these pants?"

If I had a dollar for every time I've asked or answered that question, I could retire to a tropical island. On my island, my favorite pants would always fit me—even my old jeans from college. No, even my old jeans from *high school*. There would be no cellulite on my island, and I would have sculpted thighs, slim hips, and a rock-solid bum.

It's hard not to fantasize about perfect body parts when our society equates a firm, fit body with success, beauty, power, and a happy life. Every time we turn on the TV, watch a movie, or pick up a magazine, we're bombarded by images of pencil-thin, perfectly toned models and celebrities.

Every spring, the pressure heats up even more when it seems like every women's magazine cover screams "get bikini ready!" Inside: workouts to help normal people like us get bodies like Madonna, Cameron Diaz, or Jennifer Garner. It's enough to push your envy and inadequacy buttons, big time. But consider this: There was a time when these chiseled women weren't so buff. They look great now because they worked hard to get in shape.

GET THE BUTT AND LEGS YOU WANT

If you'd like to firm up your lower half, and in the meantime, slim down, improve your coordination and balance, strengthen your legs, have more energy, walk taller, and look great in your clothes, it's never too late. Studies have shown that whether you're twenty-five, sixty-five, or even eighty-five, a regular exerciser or a beginner, you, too, can reap the benefits of a comprehensive fitness plan that includes lower-body conditioning.

Welcome to *The Little Butt & Thighs Workout Book*

You might not believe it, but you *can* diminish the appearance of cellulite, you're not saddled with your love handles forever, and you only need to do a few short workouts a week to start reshaping your rear.

How to Use This Book

The Little Butt & Thighs Workout Book will help you get started in a home exercise program designed to improve the appearance and function of your leg and buttock muscles. You'll learn how to beat cellulite, burn more calories, and perform more than sixteen strengthening and toning exercises—at home, at the gym, or anywhere you have a few feet of space.

For best results, please read the chapters in order. Before practicing any of the exercises in chapters 8 through 11, you need to prepare your body and mind. Understanding how your body moves, why posture and alignment are vital, and how to correctly apply strength training principles, will help you exercise safely and effectively.

All the exercises in this book, organized into four "miniworkouts," were carefully selected with the guidance of a licensed physical therapist and two certified personal trainers, all certified in strength training instruction. The first mini-workout contains four basic strengthening exercises, with each successive mini-workout more difficult than the last. Most of the exercises can be done without equipment. Correct technique will be the key to your success.

WHO THIS BOOK IS FOR

This book is for anyone who wants stronger, more attractive legs and a firmer butt. You'll notice that a few small sections of this book highlight women's concerns about their lower bodies. We're genetically designed to gain fat around our thighs, hips, and butts; there are no other body parts we obsess about more. But if there's a man in your life whose relaxed fit jeans aren't so relaxed anymore, you can share this book with him, too. The training guidelines and workouts are just as effective for men as they are for women.

No Buts About It

Adding lower body training to your fitness plan is easier and less time consuming than you might think—even if you're a beginner. Sure, it takes a bit of hard work, but getting rid of flabby thighs is worth it.

The exercises are easy to learn, each mini-workout takes only ten to fifteen minutes to complete, and you only have to practice them two or three times a week. Clearly written instructions guide you through each workout.

You might be surprised to realize that your greatest challenge is simply committing yourself to regular practice. I hope you'll take your time and enjoy each workout. Try not to think of exercise as a chore, but as the perfect gift for your body, a way to relieve stress, improve your health, and spend time focusing on yourself. Once you start practicing the exercises, you'll appreciate how you feel after each short workout—energized, strong, and confident. These feelings will keep you coming back for more.

Toned legs, slimmer hips, and firm buns are in your (near)

future. With discipline, patience, and consistent practice, you'll be on your way to a stronger, more functional lower body . . . that looks great in your favorite jeans (or swimsuit)!

ERIKA DILLMAN

1 | My Big Butt

Bummed Out

I never thought about the size or shape of my butt and thighs until I turned thirty-nine and realized that all of my pants were too tight. I was ten pounds overweight, small patches of rippled skin had mysteriously appeared on my inner thighs, and *I had a dimpled ass.*

How could this have happened? How could my genes have turned on me in this cruel manner? Why had clothing manufacturers started making such small pants?

My friends had no sympathy for me because I was still on the thin side for my body type, and they thought that I still looked good in my clothes. My doctor was even less concerned. "Buy bigger pants," she said.

Buy bigger pants! What's the point of going on if I can't be a size X, I thought. And what happens when I have to wear shorts or a swimsuit? (I don't mind sharing my actual pants size, but it isn't important; no matter what size or shape we are—we all want to fit into our "thin" pants.)

For the next few months, I complained about my ever-expanding butt to everyone I knew, but nobody seemed to care. I'd be waiting in line at the grocery store or watching TV, and I could actually feel my butt getting bigger. Something had to be done.

FLAB ATTACK

It's a little embarrassing to admit, but just because I'm a fitness writer and a former athlete doesn't mean my fitness plans don't get sidetracked by injuries, illness, and the chaos of having too much on my plate. And just because I'm on the thin side doesn't mean that I'm immune to cellulite or that it's easy to maintain my weight.

My Big Butt

My weight gain was my own fault. After an extended illness, during which I was unable to exercise for several months, I didn't return to my daily routine. I'd started walking two or three times a week, but I hadn't lifted a dumbbell in seven or eight months. My biggest problem: bingeing on crackers, peanuts, and corn chips every night while watching cable TV. I didn't eat much during the day, but I'd eat all night long.

Since my diet was more difficult to change, my first plan of attack was getting my muscles back into shape.

STRONGER, FIRMER

Over three weeks, I gradually increased the number and intensity of my walks until I was walking almost every day for thirty minutes at a brisk pace. (On my low-energy days, I walked slower, but tried to keep moving for forty to forty-five minutes.)

I also added three or four lower-body strength training exercises to the middle of my morning yoga routines twice a week. The strengthening exercises really worked my thigh and butt muscles; following them with some yoga stretches helped me improve my flexibility and reduce next-day soreness.

After a month, I could see muscle definition in my thighs. After six to eight weeks, my legs and butt were noticeably firmer, my legs felt stronger and more stable during movement, and my balance had improved.

These changes didn't surprise me; I knew how effective strength training was, and what it felt like to be fit. But I still got a kick out of seeing (and feeling) the results of my training. I was so happy to be active again. My walks cleared my head of stress and worry, leaving me feeling more alert and healthy. The strength training exercises energized me; after each morning workout, I felt stronger, taller, and ready to take on the day.

BINGE CONTROL

Increasing my aerobic activity and getting back into regular strength training was fairly easy for me because I enjoy exercising, I know which exercises I need to do, and I love how I feel when I'm fit. Just saying no to all of my high-fat snacks was much more difficult. So I asked for help.

I visited a registered dietitian who gave me a food plan based on my health, activity level, and caloric needs. Instead of eating most of my calories at night, I switched to eating a good breakfast in the morning and several small meals throughout the day.

As for the bingeing, I followed the advice of another dietitian I know who promotes the 80/20 principle: I eat healthy foods 80 percent of the time, and I don't beat myself up for succumbing to less healthy foods (or overeating) 20 percent of the time. I've already replaced my high-fat snacks with healthier, low-calorie alternatives like fruit and air-popped popcorn. Most important, I've learned how to readjust my portion sizes to actual serving sizes, which for many foods is only one-half to one cup.

BACK ON TRACK

Between exercising and eating the correct amount of calories for my body and activity level (not to mention watching less TV), I'm starting to lose those extra pounds I've been carrying and I'm right on track to be a size X again by the time I turn forty!

2 | The Truth About Cellulite, Fat Burning, and Weight Loss

THE BOTTOM LINE

Let's face it. Before you can get the legs you want, you have to address your cellulite situation.

We all have it. We all hate it. We spend millions every year on creams, pills, and spa treatments "guaranteed" to get rid of it. We try the latest diets and buy exercise equipment designed to help us "burn the fat," and still, most of us seem stuck with our dimpled, flabby thighs. What's a woman to do?

Get the facts about cellulite, fat burning, and weight loss.

WHAT IS CELLULITE?

Cellulite is simply a fancy word for fat. It's no different from fat in other parts of your body. When the layer of fat between your skin and muscles becomes too thick and the underlying muscles are underused, your skin takes on the shape of the fat rather than the muscle. The result: dimpled, lumpy skin.

Eighty-five to 90 percent of women have cellulite. We're genetically programmed to store fat in our hips, buttocks, and thighs. It doesn't matter if you're thin or heavy; all body types are susceptible to cellulite.

Men, on the other hand, rarely have cellulite. They tend to store fat in their abdomens. The reason they don't get dimpled thighs is also because of the way fat is connected to their skin. Women's connective tissue attaches fat to skin in a way that allows excess fat to bulge, causing dimples. Men's connective tissue has a different structure that prevents dimpling.[1]

HOW CAN I GET RID OF CELLULITE AND GET TONED LEGS?

There is no quick fix. Research has shown that herbal wraps, thigh creams, and pills don't work. Even liposuction is no guarantee against cellulite.

The only way to reduce and reshape your lower half: Lose fat and improve muscle size through exercise and diet. Regularly practicing aerobic exercise, eating a healthy diet, and monitoring your calorie consumption are vital for health and weight management. Adding strength training to your fitness plan helps you change your body composition by replacing fat with muscle. As you reduce the layer of fat between your skin and muscles and improve muscle size (don't worry, you won't get huge muscles), your skin takes on the smooth, firm shape of your muscles, giving your legs, hips, and butt a more toned appearance.

AM I TOO OLD TO HAVE TONED THIGHS AND A FIRM BUM?

You're never too old to benefit from exercise or to reduce the appearance of cellulite. In a study conducted with nursing home patients (mean age—88.5), researchers found that a six-exercise strength training program was effective in improving their strength, flexibility, and body composition.[2]

It's important to stay active no matter how old you are. Starting sometime between thirty and thirty-five, both muscle and bone begin to break down as part of the natural aging process. The average woman loses 5 pounds of muscle (men lose 7) and gains 15 pounds (men gain 17) of fat every decade —and loses 1 percent of her bone mass every year. After menopause, a woman can lose 10 pounds of muscle a decade and 2 to 2½ percent bone loss every year.[3] *Unless*, that is, she exercises regularly and doesn't consume more calories than she needs.

HOW DO I LOSE THOSE EXTRA POUNDS AND KEEP THEM OFF?

If you want to lose weight, you have to burn off more calories than you consume to create a calorie deficit. To maintain your weight, you need to be active enough to burn off the calories you eat. Extra calories, whether they come from carbs, protein, or fat, are stored as fat.

Dieting alone is not effective in changing your body composition because as you lose fat, you also lose muscle tissue. Consistent strength training is the only way to prevent muscle loss and to reshape your muscles.

HOW MANY CALORIES DO I NEED?

Your daily caloric needs are based on your age, gender, size, activity levels, and weight goals. The best person to determine your caloric needs is a registered dietitian (someone with an R.D. after her or his name), who can take all your health and genetic factors into account.

However, for a quick estimate, you can determine an approximate figure by calculating your *resting metabolic rate* (also called *basal metabolic rate*),[4] or, the base number of calories your body needs at rest. Once you have this number, you can figure out how many calories you need to fuel all of your daily activities. (See "Calculating Your Daily Caloric Needs," page 18.)

Knowing your caloric needs helps you plan your eating and activities according to your weight control and fitness goals. Remember, the dietary information on food labels is based on the 2,000-calorie daily intake associated with the traditional food pyramid designed by the U.S. Department of Agriculture. You may need to adjust serving sizes to fit your caloric needs.

You might be tempted to drastically reduce your caloric intake to lose weight, but keep in mind that consuming fewer than 10 calories per pound of weight actually slows your metabolism. (**Caution:** Extremely low-calorie diets are not healthy and can be dangerous. According to the National Institutes of Health, women should consume at least 1,200 calories a day and men should consume at least 1,500 calories a day. Consult your doctor if you are interested in an extremely low-calorie diet.)[5]

CALCULATING YOUR DAILY CALORIC NEEDS

1. Multiply your weight (in pounds) by 10 calories per pound (11 for men) to determine your resting metabolic rate.

Example: Alice is a 140-pound woman. Her resting metabolic rate is 1,400 calories. To keep her heart pumping, her lungs exchanging new air for stale air, and all of her other organs working, she needs to eat 1,400 calories a day.

Next, calculate how many calories you need each day to fuel all of your activities.

2. Multiply your *resting metabolic rate* by the appropriate activity level (.20, .30, .40, or .50) to determine your activity calories.

    .20 no exercise, sedentary lifestyle
    .30 exercise occasionally
    .40 exercise regularly (3x/week for 30 minutes or more)
    .50 exercise most days, train for a sport, or have a physically demanding job

Example: Alice is moderately active; she swims 3 times a week and lifts weights 2 times a week. 1,400 × .40 = 560. Alice needs 560 calories to fuel all her activities.

Now, factor in the calories your body uses to digest your meals.

3. Multiply the sum of your resting metabolic rate and activity caloric needs by .1 to determine your digestion calories.

Example: Alice needs (1,400 + 560) × .1 = 196 calories for digestion.

Finally, add up all of your calories to determine your total daily caloric needs.

4. Add your resting metabolic rate, your activity calories, and your digestion calories for your total daily calories.

Example: Alice needs 1,400 + 560 + 196 = 2,156 calories a day to adequately fuel her body.

You can use the charts in the back of the book to find out estimated caloric needs for men and women, as well as to see how many calories you can burn in different types of daily, recreational, and athletic activities. (See Appendix B, page 157.)

Don't forget, if your activity levels change, you need to alter your caloric intake accordingly. Most important, avoid falling into the "I just exercised so I can eat anything I want" trap. Even if you exercise vigorously enough to burn off 300 to 400 calories in one workout, you don't get a free pass to eat a pint of Ben & Jerry's (1,200 calories!) that evening. Strive for moderate eating and regular exercise.

SHOULD I STOP EATING FATS AND CARBOHYDRATES?

Fats and carbohydrates don't necessarily make you fat. Eating more calories than you burn off does. Your body needs some fat to function optimally. A simple rule of thumb: Reduce or eliminate from your diet cholesterol-raising saturated fats (found in dairy foods, red meat, chocolate, and coconut oil) and trans fats (found in deep-fried foods, such processed foods as crackers and cookies, and fast-food products), replacing them with adequate serving sizes of healthy monounsaturated fats (found in olive oil, peanut butter, and avocado) and polyunsaturated fats (found in fish, soybeans, and corn) that lower cholesterol levels.[6]

The Truth About Cellulite, Fat Burning, and Weight Loss

As for carbs, the only reason they're getting a bad rap is because people eat too many of the wrong types of carbs (e.g., white bread, pasta, cookies, white rice, crackers, potatoes), thus missing out on the nutrients they need and consuming too many calories.

You don't need to eliminate carbs from your diet—but rather, switch to whole grain products. Look for products made from whole wheat, and avoid enriched, bleached flour. Also, pay attention to serving sizes (which are often only one-half to one cup), and indulge in fruits and vegetables (don't forget, they provide carbs, too). Instead of eating a massive bowl of pasta topped with a few vegetables, eat a small amount of whole grain or soy pasta topped with a generous portion of vegetables.

Start shopping for food the same way you'd shop for a luxury car or a computer—ask questions, read the labels, and buy the best products you can afford. If you want your body to function optimally, feed it the best food available. I highly recommend reading *Eat, Drink, and Be Healthy* by Harvard Medical School's Walter C. Willett, M.D., an easy-to-read book that explains how to reorganize the traditional food pyramid for healthier eating.

WHAT'S THE BEST DIET FOR WEIGHT LOSS OR WEIGHT CONTROL?

Despite the promises of best-selling diet books, there is no "best" diet. In fact, 90 to 95 percent of women aren't successful at losing weight or maintaining weight loss through dieting because as soon as they stop restricting their food intake, they regain the weight they've lost.[7]

Rather than trying fad diets and depriving yourself of your favorite foods, work with a registered dietitian who can develop a realistic eating plan for you based on your daily caloric needs.

For the price of two or three diet books, you'll get an eating plan that includes a variety of healthy foods, sample menus, and low-fat alternatives to your favorite high-fat snacks. Your nutritionist can also teach you how to readjust portion sizes to actual serving sizes (most of us are so used to eating massive portions that we don't even realize how many extra calories we consume each meal) and how to spread out your caloric intake throughout the day to maximize your energy levels. (For example, eating five or six small meals throughout the day is a great way to meet your daily nutritional requirements, add variety to your diet, and control calories.)

———

Making gradual lifestyle changes that promote healthier eating and regular exercise is an effective way to lose and control your weight. Sticking to healthy habits will help you reach and maintain your goals over the long haul. (See Resources, page 163, for suggested reading on diet and nutrition.)

WHAT'S THE BEST WAY TO BURN FAT?

You've probably heard a lot about the "fat burning zone," a period of time during low-intensity exercises, such as walking or hiking, at which your body begins to burn fat as fuel. Even cardio machines have settings for "fat-burning" workouts. Unfortunately, these terms can be very misleading, and it's actually quite difficult for the average person to accurately calculate her "zone."

Rather than focusing on fat, keep it simple—think about total calories burned in a given activity. After all, that's the currency which with you're dealing—you gain calories from eating, you burn calories from exercising.

Your body uses both carbohydrates (in the form of glycogen, a sugar) and fat for fuel. The percentages of fat or carbohy-

———

drates "burned" in any given activity depends on your size, the activity, and the length and intensity of your workout. Here's how it works: You have thirty minutes to run or walk. If you go for a walk, you'll burn a higher percentage of fat calories than you will running for thirty minutes. But, running is a high-intensity exercise that burns more total calories in the same amount of time, so you'll end up burning more fat calories, too.

The bottom line: A calorie is a calorie. Let your body worry about what type of fuel it burns. You just need to keep moving.

TAKE ACTION

Maybe you just need a bit of exercise to tone up, or maybe you also want to lose ten or fifteen pounds. Whatever your goal, you can start now. You're already on track for positive change by learning more about your body in these preliminary chapters.

3 | Meet Your Muscles

BASIC ANATOMY AND PHYSIOLOGY

You're always asking your muscles to work for *you*, but what do you really know about *them* and what they need to function optimally?

Before you strengthen and reshape your lower-body muscles, it's a good idea to know where they're located and how they function.

MOVERS AND STABILIZERS

Like all skeletal muscles, your lower-body muscles work alone and synergistically (i.e., in conjunction with other muscles) to move your body, to move individual body parts, and to maintain posture.

You're probably very familiar with your "quads" (front of thigh), hamstrings (back of thigh), and "glutes" (butt) muscles—they're the big muscles, called primary movers, that help you walk, run, jump, squat, and climb stairs. They're also the lower-body equivalent of the biceps, the "show me your muscle" muscles that when toned, give you that lean, cut look. *(See Figure 3.1, the Muscle Map, for general locations of the major lower-body muscles.)*

You may be less familiar with the *secondary movers,* smaller muscles that assist with movement, and the *stabilizers,* even smaller muscles, usually located around joints, that hold one body part in place while another body part moves.

While these classifications present a very simplified view of muscle function, it's helpful to keep in mind that every movement you make requires a variety of muscles to perform their jobs correctly.

Meet Your Muscles

Figure 3.1
Muscle Map

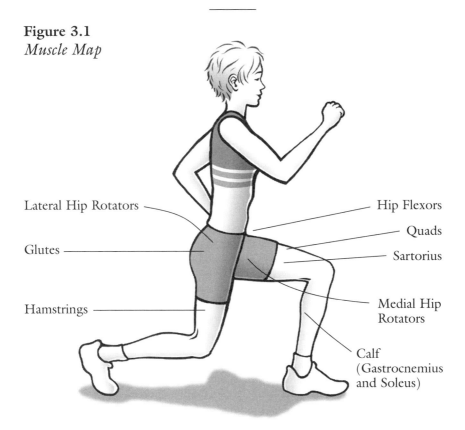

Lateral Hip Rotators

Glutes

Hamstrings

Hip Flexors

Quads

Sartorius

Medial Hip Rotators

Calf (Gastrocnemius and Soleus)

RESTORING BALANCE

When it comes to lower-body conditioning, it's important to work all of the muscles involved in hip and leg movements. Most people have muscle imbalances throughout their bodies, where some muscles are too weak to adequately perform their designated functions and others are overused in compensation. This type of imbalance increases injury risk to joints, muscles, bones, and connective tissues.

Practicing the lower-body exercises in this book will help you strengthen all the muscles involved in lower-body movements—large and small, movers and stabilizers—restoring balanced strength, coordination, and muscle tone.

The Muscle Function Chart on pages 30–31, will help you learn more about the primary functions of the major lower body muscles.

PUTTING YOUR MUSCLES TO WORK

As you can see, your lower-body muscles have many responsibilities, primarily, supporting and moving your legs and pelvis.

Meet Your Muscles

(They also play an important role in posture.) Understanding the basic anatomy and physiology of your thighs, hips, and butt will improve your mind-body awareness, helping you visualize your muscles at work and maintain your focus during each exercise.

THE LITTLE BUTT & THIGHS WORKOUT BOOK

MUSCLE FUNCTION CHART			
Muscle Location	**Muscle Name**	**Functions/ Characteristics**	**Exercises That Work Muscle(s)**
Front of thigh	Quadriceps ("quads")	Knee extension (straightens leg).	Squats, Lunges
Back of thigh	Hamstrings	Knee flexion (bends leg); hip extension (moves thigh behind body); lateral thigh rotation (rotates thigh away from center of body).	Squats, Lunges
Inner thigh	Sartorius	Hip flexion (moves thigh in front of body); assists in knee flexion (bends leg) and lateral knee rotation (rotates knee toward center of body). Longest muscle in the body.	Squats, Lunges
Buttocks/ back of hips	Gluteals ("glutes") (gluteus maximus, gluteus minimus, gluteus medius)	Hip extension, flexion, lateral and medial rotation of hip, abduction (moves thigh away from center of body); moves and stabilizes pelvis. The gluteus maximus is the largest, and one of the strongest, muscles in the body.	Bridges, Bent-Leg Crossover, Hydrant, Squats, Lunges

Meet Your Muscles

Muscle Location	Muscle Name	Functions/ Characteristics	Exercises That Work Muscle(s)
Front of hips	Hip flexors (psoas, iliacus, tensor fasciae latae)	Hip flexion, medial and lateral rotation of hip, adduction (moves thigh toward center of body). Assists with pelvic movement and stability.	4-Way Hip Motion with Band
Buttocks/ sides of hips	Lateral hip rotators	Assist gluteus maximus in hip rotation (rotates thigh away from center of the body).	Side Plank with Leg Lift
Inner thigh	Medial hip rotators	Rotates thigh toward the center of the body.	Bent-Leg Crossover
Calf	Gastrocnemius, soleus	Knee extension (straightens leg); plantar flexion of ankle (helps foot push off against ground when walking or running).	Lunges

A note about hips: When you practice the exercises (and stretches), you'll need to know how to locate your hips. They're not just where your pants sit, but two ball-and-socket joints surrounded by muscles on each side of your pelvis. Think of your hips as the front, back, and outer sides of your pelvis.

Sources: Blandine Calais-Germain. *Anatomy of Movement.* Eastland Press (Seattle, WA), 1993; Kurt, Mike, and Brett Brungardt. *The Complete Book of Butt and Legs.* Villard Books (New York), 1995; Frédéric Devalier. *Strength Training Anatomy.* Human Kinetics (Champaign, IL), 2001.

4 | How to Get Toned Legs and a Firm Butt

REDUCE, RESHAPE, RECHARGE

Strength training is the key to changing your body composition. It's also one of the best ways to recharge your metabolism, helping you manage or lose weight.

BOOSTING METABOLISM

Many people don't realize that their muscles play a vital role in metabolism. The more muscle mass you have, the higher your metabolism and the more calories you burn. That's why men sometimes seem to have an easier time losing weight than women by reducing calories alone; they have more muscle mass for burning calories. Women, on the other hand, often need to change their metabolism with exercise if they want to lose weight. When it comes to changing shape, both men and women need strength training.

In a healthy body, muscle tissue should take up most of the space between your skin and bones. As you age, or if you're inactive, your muscles atrophy (i.e., get smaller), and you gain fat that eventually takes up more space than your muscles. *(See Figure 4.1.)* With smaller muscles, your metabolism drops and

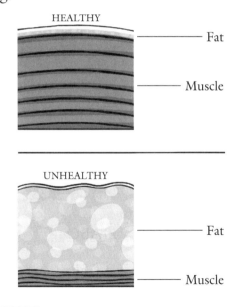

HEALTHY

Fat

Muscle

UNHEALTHY

Fat

Muscle

Figure 4.1
Body Composition

you don't burn as many calories. When you consider that the lower-body muscles are some of the largest muscles in your body, you're missing out on a lot of calorie-burning if you don't keep them in shape.

It is possible to lose weight and reduce the fat layer between your skin and muscles through calorie reduction, aerobic exercise, or a combination of the two, but both methods cause muscle tissue loss along with the fat loss. Strength training is the best way to restore healthy body composition, improve muscle strength and shape, and in turn, significantly boost your metabolism.

THE TRIPLE BURN

Strength training helps your body burn more calories at rest and during activity in three ways. First, you burn calories during your strength training session. Next, your metabolism stays elevated for an hour or two after a strength training session, during which time you burn 25 percent of the calories you burned during your workout. Finally, once you've trained long enough to add three pounds of muscle, you increase your resting metabolic rate by 7 percent, burning an additional 90 to 120 calories a day (each additional pound of muscle added burns between 30 and 40 calories a day).[1]

Therefore, if you weigh 140 pounds and you strength-train for 30 minutes (including upper- and lower-body exercises), you'll burn 218 calories. In the 2 hours after your workout, you'll burn an additional 54 calories. And once you've gained 3 pounds of muscle mass (which takes 2 or 3 months), you'll burn an additional 98 calories a day. That's a total of 370 calories burned for every day you strength-train. Not bad for 30 minutes of work.

Practice three strength training workouts a week, and you'll burn 1,110 calories per week. Add two 30-minute walks at a brisk pace (2 × 185) and 30 minutes of swimming (281), and you'll burn an additional 651 calories that week for a total of 1,761 calories. That's enough activity to lose half a pound in a week.

POUND FOR POUND

For safety and long-term success, dietitians generally recommend losing no more than 1 pound a week. Depending on how active you want to be, you can lose a pound a week, or pursue a more reasonable goal: losing two to three pounds a month.

There are 3,500 calories in a pound; creating a 3,500-calorie deficit is the only way to lose 1 pound. As you read above, a 140-pound person can burn 1,761 calories a week practicing strength training three times a week and aerobic exercise three times a week. If that person also cuts 500 calories from her or his diet each week (for example, cutting out two lattes a week),[2] the weekly calorie deficit dips to 2,261. At the end of the month, your calorie deficit equals a 2½-pound weight loss. That puts you on track to lose 15 pounds in six months just by adding some activity, consuming only the calories you need, and cutting out a few high-fat snacks.

It's helpful to keep in mind that your body decides where fat loss occurs. Unfortunately, you can't "spot reduce" by exercising specific body parts. However, strength training will tone specific body parts, and as you lose weight throughout your body, your tone will become more visible.

FIRM UP, SLIM DOWN

It may seem strange to build muscles to get smaller or thinner, but remember, your goal is restoring a healthy body composition, where muscles occupy most of the space between your skin and bones. You'll be replacing unhealthy amounts of fat with healthy, calorie-burning muscle.

Of course, you want to achieve and maintain a healthy weight, but your ratio of fat to muscle is also critical in determining your shape and keeping you healthy. Being overweight and having too much body fat is associated with a variety of health problems, such as heart disease, stroke, diabetes, and some types of cancer.

Don't be alarmed if, after several weeks of training, you look better and your clothes fit better, but your weight doesn't change as much as you think it should. Muscle weighs more than fat, so if you lose ten pounds of fat and gain two to three pounds of muscle, you'll only notice a seven- to eight-pound weight loss even if you've trimmed down. It's more important to be slimmer, stronger, healthy, and in shape than obsess about a number on the scale.

BUILDING A STRONG FOUNDATION

Strength training isn't just about your appearance; it's an important element of health and fitness. You've probably never thought about "training" to be in shape for your daily life. But you should.

Your legs are your body's foundation. They need to be strong enough to support your body in all of its daily activities. Even if you regularly practice moderate-intensity weight-bearing activities (such as hiking, walking, running) for cardio-vascular fitness and muscle endurance, you still need strength training to significantly improve muscle strength, size, and shape.

The best way to strengthen and tone your lower half is by practicing compound, multi-joint exercises (i.e., exercises that involve several muscles and more than one joint). These exercises train large muscles, as well as smaller, supportive muscles, through a chain of movement, and work muscles in opposing pairs (e.g., the muscles that straighten your leg and the muscles that bend your leg), building balanced strength throughout the body.

Weight-bearing compound exercises, such as the squat (page

72) and the lunge (page 75), challenge your leg, hip, and butt muscles to work together in supporting your body weight during movement. This type of training is called "functional training."

Functional exercises, or exercises that mimic everyday movements, retrain your muscles, connective tissues, and nervous system to function optimally, helping you develop an integrated strength that translates into better balance, more graceful movements, stronger joints, improved posture, and greater strength and endurance.

RESIZING YOUR THIGHS

If you're not exactly sure what strength training is or how it works, here's a brief explanation:

Strength training exercises challenge your muscles to lift or move an amount of weight (also referred to as resistance) that is heavier than they're used to handling. By progressively "overloading" your muscles, or, asking your muscles to lift more weight, you train them to adapt to each new workload. With each challenge, individual muscle fibers enlarge and blood vessels and nerves serving muscles become more efficient at their jobs. The results: Your muscles get more oxygen from your blood (you get more energy); your nervous system becomes more adept at telling your muscles what to do (your coordination and balance improve); and your muscles get stronger and bigger (your strength, endurance, and muscle tone improve). (**Note:** A general strength training program won't produce bulging muscles, especially in women, who lack sufficient quantities of the male hormone testosterone, to "bulk up.")

Strength training exercises can be done with weights, such as dumbbells or barbells; on weight machines found at health clubs; with stability balls and rubber tubing; or using your own body as resistance. Most of the exercises in this book can be practiced without equipment.

5 | Exercise Guidelines

STRONGER, SLIMMER BY DESIGN

Great legs and a firm butt are the results of consistent training.

The mini-workouts in this book form the core of your lower-body shape-up plan. For best results, and to maintain a healthy, balanced body, you'll need to include a variety of exercises in your weekly fitness program, such as upper-body strength training, aerobic activity, and flexibility exercises.

Understanding some basic exercise guidelines will help you plan your workouts.

GUIDELINES: YOUR EXERCISE PLAN

Although each mini-workout includes instructions, it's helpful to know the guidelines that were used to design them so that you can begin to plan your own workouts as you learn more exercises.

The following guidelines are based on recommendations by such health and fitness organizations as the National Strength and Conditioning Association (NSCA) and the American College of Sports Medicine (ACSM).

Reps, Sets, and Resistance

"Reps" are repetitions or the number of times you perform an exercise, and sets are groups of reps. *Resistance* refers to the amount of weight you lift or work against. In the weight-free exercises in this book, you'll be using your own body weight as resistance.

To improve muscle size, do 1 to 3 sets of 8 to 10 reps. Beginners can start with 1 set. (Research has shown that 1 set of each exercise is adequate for improving strength. However, as you progress, you'll want to add more sets to keep your body challenged.)[1]

You might find that many of the exercises are quite challenging, and that you are unable to perform 8 reps. That's fine. In fact, once you can easily perform 10 reps of an exercise, you need to add resistance (by modifying the exercise or by using weights) in order to keep the exercise challenging enough that you reach muscle fatigue by 8 reps. In this case, more is not better. Once you can do 10, 12, or 15 reps of an exercise, your efforts are actually affecting muscle endurance more than size or strength. Practicing within the 8 to 10 rep muscle-building range will help you improve size and strength.

Keep in mind: It's better to do 3 or 4 reps in correct form than 8 to 10 in bad form.

Your Plan: 1 to 3 sets of 8 to 10 reps.

Frequency, Duration

Practice lower-body strength training two or three times a week, with at least one or two days between workouts. Beginners can improve with just two workouts a week, but as your body adapts to training, you might want to add another workout to increase the intensity. Each mini-workout takes only ten to fifteen minutes to perform.

Your Plan: 2 to 3 workouts per week.

Warm Up, Cool Down

Before your workout, spend at least five minutes warming up your muscles with light aerobic exercise such as riding a stationary bike or taking a short walk. You'll notice pretty quickly that lower-body training can leave your muscles tight, especially your hamstrings and glutes, so you'll need to do at least five to ten minutes of stretching after your workout. Research has shown that including stretching in strength training workouts improves muscle strength, range of motion, and flexibility.[2]

You can also stretch after each exercise. For example, after an exercise that works your hamstrings, do a hamstring stretch before moving on to the next exercise. There are a few stretches in the back of the book (Appendix A, page 145) to get you started, but for more complete information on stretching, please check the resources listed in the back of the book or consult a personal trainer.

Your Plan: 5 to 10 minutes of aerobic warm-up and at least 5 to 10 minutes of stretching to cool down.

Pacing, Intensity, and Interest

Exercise at a steady, efficient pace in order to maintain intensity. Ideally, rest for thirty seconds between sets. You may need to rest for sixty to ninety seconds when you begin, but try to pick up the pace a bit as you get more proficient with each exercise. You don't have to hurry; just keep moving.

Changing your routine every six to eight weeks helps you continue making progress and keeps you interested in your training. Here are a few ways to maintain and increase the intensity of your workouts: Progress to the next mini-workout, supplement your current routine with exercises from other mini-workouts, take shorter rest breaks between exercises, or change the order in which you practice the exercises. If you want to keep improving tone and strength, practice exercises that cause fatigue by 8 reps (you can do this by increasing resistance and adding more sets).

When it comes to changing your body composition, slow and steady wins the race. Only change one variable at a time, and only increase resistance in small increments (one to three pounds). With four mini-workouts, totaling 16 exercises, you'll have more than enough to do for many months.

Your Plan: Revamp your workout every 6 to 8 weeks.

Rest and Recovery

Rest is just as important as exercise. Your muscles need at least forty-eight hours to recover from a strength training workout. If you want to exercise every day, do lower-body strength training one day, and upper-body training the next. It's okay to train if you're a little bit sore, but if you've overdone it and your muscles hurt, wait a day or two longer before your next strength training session.

THE BIG PICTURE

Getting the legs and butt you want is a worthy goal, but don't forget: For overall health and fitness, you need to keep your body active, toned, and flexible with a variety of exercises, including:

- *Aerobic exercise.* Health and fitness organizations recommend 30 to 60 minutes of moderately paced aerobic exercise (such as walking, running, riding a bicycle, swimming, inline skating, and other activities that work the body's largest muscles) most days of the week. Regular aerobic exercise is important for maintaining cardiovascular health, improving blood pressure and cholesterol levels, burning calories, controlling weight, providing protection from disease, and reducing anxiety and depression.

    The recommended amount of exercise is based on levels of activity that health experts believe provide health benefits. You may need more or less than the recommended guidelines depending on your health and fitness goals. A beginner or an older adult will start off with a different exercise plan than an athlete training for competition or someone trying to lose a significant amount of weight.

- *Upper-body strength training.* In order to build balanced strength throughout the body, and for maximum calorie burning, your fitness plan should also include two or three strength training workouts a week that work muscles in the torso and upper body. Each mini-workout in this book represents almost half of a complete strength training workout, and takes only 10 to 15 minutes to complete. Adding upper body moves adds about 10 to 20 minutes to your workout, depending on the types of exercises you practice and on how many sets you do. If you prefer, alternate practicing upper- and lower-body exercises on consecutive days.
- *Flexibility exercises.* Practice flexibility exercises such as stretching and yoga a few times a week to maintain muscle suppleness, good posture, and alignment.

This may sound like a lot of activity, but once you break it down into small, almost daily workouts, you'll see that in the time it takes you to watch one TV sitcom a day, you can improve your muscle strength and tone, boost your metabolism, improve your energy levels, and get a healthier, more attractive body.

If you'd like to learn more about upper-body and core strength training exercises as well as flexibility exercises, consult *The Little Strength Training Book*, *The Little Abs Workout Book*, and *The Little Yoga Book*.

6 | Essential Training Techniques

TIPS FOR SUCCESS

The key to your success in reshaping your lower body is correct form.

Just as you use a special technique to lift a heavy box, you'll be applying similar ergonomic principles to each exercise. Practicing good body mechanics helps you retrain your muscles to work in healthy movement patterns, protecting you from injury, building functional strength, and improving muscle tone.

YOU'RE ONLY AS HEALTHY AS YOUR SPINE

Good posture helps you look healthy, strong, and confident. It's also essential for maintaining correct alignment throughout your body.

So many of us spend our days sitting at desks or in cars, slouching into little question marks. Then at the end of the day, we try to lift our groceries into our cars or play sports, and wonder why we have sore backs and necks.

Take a minute now, and see what good posture feels like.

GOOD POSTURE FROM THE BOTTOM UP

Stand Firm

Plant your feet firmly on the floor, about hips-width apart. Keep your legs straight, but don't lock your knees. Gently engage your thigh muscles, pulling up your kneecaps.

Use Your Abs

Pull your abdominal muscles up and in toward your spine to help maintain neutral spine and correct pelvic and spinal alignment in the lower back.

Continued . . .

Lift Your Chest

Slightly raise your chest to take the slouch out of your mid-back.

Relax Your Shoulders

Allow your shoulders to relax, resting down and away from your ears, and your arms to hang at your sides.

Stand Tall

Imagine that there's a string running vertically through the center of your body and out the top of your head *and* that someone much taller than you is gently pulling up on that string. Let your body relax into alignment. Hold your head high, keep your neck straight, long, relaxed, and look straight ahead with your chin parallel to the floor.

You'll notice that when your body is correctly aligned your ears, shoulders, hips, knees, and ankles form a straight line—and you can breathe easier because your internal organs are no longer scrunched together. Try maintaining this posture throughout the day, whether sitting or standing.

POSTURE IN ACTION

It's more difficult to maintain your posture and alignment during movement, but it's even more important. If your legs and postural muscles aren't strong enough to hold your body upright, you're going to have a pretty tough time hiking with a backpack, putting enough power into your kicking leg to boot a soccer ball down the field, or even squatting to do the lifting required in many household chores. Your body is strongest, and your muscles and joints most able to function optimally, when you're correctly aligned.

PRACTICE CORRECT FORM

As you read in chapter 4, your lower-body muscles play an important role in posture by moving and supporting the pelvis. In order to restore balanced strength and optimal functioning to your body, always pay attention to your form during lower-body exercises (or any exercises). Exercising in poor posture simply reinforces bad body mechanics. All of the exercise instructions in this book contain technique tips to remind you to move in correct alignment.

Maintaining correct alignment while exercising also helps prevent injuries. Many people mistakenly believe that some types of exercise are harmful to their backs (or knees) because they've injured themselves in the past. What they don't realize is that using correct body mechanics will help them exercise without pain.

Before you practice the exercises, remember to protect your back. Don't arch your lower back or slouch. If you need to move your torso, bend at your hips (keeping your chest up will help you maintain correct posture even when

Figure 6.1 *The Spine*

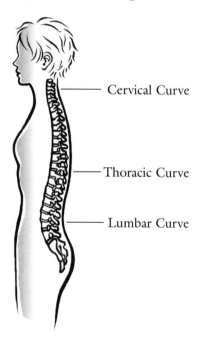

Cervical Curve

Thoracic Curve

Lumbar Curve

moving or bending forward). Most important: Straight (whether you're talking about backs, arms, or legs) never means rigid. As you can see in Figure 6.1, your spine, in correct posture, has three natural curves.

NEUTRAL SPINE

If you've taken a yoga, Pilates, or exercise class, or read a fitness magazine, you might be familiar with the term "neutral spine," which refers to your spine's optimal alignment for weight bearing. Maintaining neutral spine throughout the day, and especially during activity, helps you maintain correct posture, protecting your lower back.

Try this simple floor exercise to find neutral spine:

- Lie on your back with your feet flat on the floor, heels about 9 to 12 inches in front of buttocks.
- Using your abdominal muscles, slowly and gently roll your pelvis backward, pressing your lower back into the floor.
- Next, using your lower-back muscles, slowly and gently roll

your pelvis forward, creating an arch between your lower back and the floor. Return to starting position.

• Neutral spine is the spinal position in between these two positions.

As you can see in this exercise, your spinal alignment is linked to your pelvic alignment. Another way to check in with your posture while in a standing position is to imagine that your pelvis is a large bowl of water that's sitting on a stable platform (in fact, the word *pelvis* means "basin"); as long as your pelvis is aligned you won't spill the water.[1] This isn't to say that you need to hold your body in a rigid position; good posture isn't static, but a fluid collaboration of your spine, pelvis, and muscles within a small range of positions.

USE YOUR ABS

Your abdominal muscles play a vital role in pelvic alignment. They're also the power center of your body, involved in every movement you make. Try hitting a tennis ball with a racquet or kicking a soccer ball; without your abs, you won't put much power behind your punch, you'll have a harder time balancing, and you'll be putting your lower back at risk of injury.

Before you perform any of the strengthening exercises in this book, you'll be instructed to "pull your abs up and in toward your spine" and reminded to "maintain abs to spine." Some fitness instructors use the term "navel to spine," but I prefer a bit more detailed instruction so that you remember two critical aspects of this technique:

1. Pulling up on your abs engages all four layers of your abdominal muscles to work together, so that when you pull them in toward the spine, they form a corset of protection for your spine.
2. You want your abs to protect the length of your lower spine, not just the point beneath your belly button. If at the same time you can also activate the muscles in your pelvic floor (i.e., perform a Kegel exercise) and lower back, you'll provide your spine with the protection it needs.

Think of "pulling your abs up and in toward your spine" as zipping up your abdomen from your pubic bone to your navel.

CONTROL AND FORM

Sometimes it's difficult to focus when all you can think about is the next item on your "to-do" list. Try taking your time when exercising so that you adequately prepare for and correctly perform each exercise.

Swaying and jerky movements are okay on the dance floor, but check them at the door during strength training workouts. Instead, use slow, controlled movements during both phases of the exercises (i.e., the *concentric phase*—where you exert your muscles for the first time or lift a weight, and the *eccentric phase*—when you return to the starting position or lower a weight). You're striving for grace and power, smoothly moving through each exercise and on to the next. As a general rule, exhale for two seconds during the lifting phase and inhale for four seconds as you return to the starting position. The exceptions to this rule: squats and lunges, where you'll be inhaling as you lower your body and exhaling as you raise it. Each exercise will include breathing instructions.

Pay close attention to the instructions, and read them more than once before you try each exercise so that you have a clear understanding of how to maintain posture and align body parts, as well as the type of movement you'll be making. Concentrate on your movement, and visualize your muscles at work to boost your mind-body awareness, maintain your balance, and stay focused.

LISTEN TO YOUR BODY

It's okay to feel a bit sore following a workout, but you should never feel sharp or stabbing pain when exercising. If you feel pain, dizziness, or any other unpleasant sensation, stop exercising and consult your doctor.

The exercises in this book are safe for healthy adults when practiced correctly. Some people are wary of practicing squats and lunges (there are several in this book; they're the most effective thigh and butt toners) because they're afraid of injuring their knees. However, in most cases, squats and lunges are only bad for your knees if practiced incorrectly (or if you have an injury, biomechanical problem, or mobility issue that makes these exercises unsuitable for you). If you're not sure you can do these exercises, ask your doctor, who may recommend that you work with a physical therapist who can modify these exercises to suit your needs. If you are unable to practice squats or lunges, there are still plenty of exercises in this book to help you strengthen and reshape your lower body.

When it comes to your joints, the expression "use it or lose it" really applies. If you want to continue bending your knees into old age and performing such basic daily tasks as sitting down in and getting up from a chair, you need to have strong legs that are trained to support your body weight, especially when bending, squatting, or balancing on one foot.

DON'T FORGET AIR AND WATER

It's easy to become so wrapped up in practicing each exercise that you forget to breathe. Holding your breath during strength training can be harmful and can raise your blood pressure. Instead, use your breath to help facilitate each movement, exhaling during the exertion phase and inhaling during the pre- or post-exertion phases. *Always* breathe during the pause phases of each exercise.

Essential Training Techniques

By the time you feel thirsty, you're already dehydrated. There's no need to drown yourself; just aim for eight glasses of water a day. Have a glass before your workout and another afterward.

7 | Getting Started

CHANGING YOUR SHAPE

Congratulations! By reading to this point, you've already taken a big step toward a more toned and functional lower body. Change is never simple, especially when it involves food and exercise. So give yourself some credit for committing to your reshaping plan. Remember, discipline and patience will probably challenge you more than the physical exercises.

All you need to do now is review the following short checklist to make sure you're totally prepared to begin your first mini-workout.

Getting Started

Before You Begin

Here are a few essentials you need before you begin:

- *Comfortable workout clothes.* You can wear form-fitting exercise gear or shorts and a T-shirt—whatever allows you to move freely. Also, wear stable athletic shoes that provide adequate support during side-to-side movements.
- *A doctor's "okay."* Before beginning any exercise program, it's wise to consult a doctor, especially if you have knee, back, or neck problems; are pregnant; or have a known medical condition. The exercises here are appropriate for people of all ages and skill levels, but only you and your doctor can determine which exercises suit your individual needs.
- *Assistance.* Reading this book is an excellent way to get started in a lower-body training program, but don't be afraid to ask for help if you need it. Physical therapists and certified personal trainers can teach you how to perform (and to adapt) the lower-body moves in this book. Learning correct form is worth the expense of one ($35–$75) or two sessions with a fitness professional. Your doctor can refer you to a

physical therapist (check to see if your insurance will pay for the visit), or you can work with a certified personal trainer (or a certified strength and conditioning specialist).

- *Equipment.* The majority of the exercises can be done without any equipment. For variety, and to challenge your muscles in new ways, you'll utilize rubber exercise bands and tubing or a stability ball in a few exercises. You may also want to use dumbbells or a weighted vest to modify some exercises. (For specific guidelines on rubber exercise bands and stability balls, see pages 89 and 123 in Workout Two and Workout Four, respectively.)

- *Set goals.* If you're reading this book your goals probably include firming your flabby thighs and reducing the appearance of butt dimples. Maybe you'd also like to prepare your legs for an upcoming biking trip. Maybe your goal is simply making the time to do two lower-body workouts a week. Whatever you'd like to achieve, it's helpful to set both short- and long-term goals to keep you focused on your training.

You'll be most successful if your goals are realistic and attainable. Trying to lose 10 or 20 pounds in one month or make the Olympic team will just frustrate and discourage you.

But losing 1 to 4 pounds a month and having your clothes fit better in 3 to 4 months (just in time for your birthday, anniversary, or class reunion) are definitely achievable.

• *Be kind to yourself.* As you proceed, stay disciplined, but be patient with yourself. Your body didn't get where it is overnight, and you won't be able to change it overnight. Don't abandon all hope if you stop exercising for a few days or weeks; everyone's fitness plans get derailed now and then. Simply start over at the beginning, and try to get back into a regular exercise schedule.

WHAT TO EXPECT

It's common to feel stronger and energized after just one workout; this feeling will keep you motivated to stick with your fitness plan. During the first four to six weeks of training your muscles and nerves go through an adaptation phase where they become more proficient at making the movements in each exercise. This "retraining" period helps lay the foundation for real change.

After six to eight weeks, you'll start noticing changes. You'll feel stronger, your legs will feel firmer, and your balance will improve. You'll also have more energy, you'll be able to walk or run farther before your legs feel tired, and you'll have an easier time performing everyday chores. At this point, you'll also be able to increase the intensity of your mini-workouts by exercising more frequently, adding more exercises to your routine, or practicing more challenging exercises. If you train consistently, after three months you'll gain two or three pounds of muscle, which in turn will help your body burn more calories, even at rest.

In a study of beginning exercisers, regular strength training (25-minute workouts, two to three times a week, for 8 to 12 weeks) helped female participants gain an average of 2 pounds of muscle, lose an average of 4 pounds of fat, and improve muscle strength by 40 percent. Men gained an average of 4 pounds of muscle, lost 7 pounds of fat, and improved strength by 55 percent.[1]

Evaluating Your Progress

In addition to the functional results just mentioned, here are a few more ways to evaluate your progress:

- Look in the mirror to see if you've slimmed down (you might want to take before and after photos).
- Measure your thighs, hips, and butt before you begin and after three months of training—losing one half to one inch is a significant accomplishment.
- Pay attention to how your clothes fit (you should notice a bit more room in those almost-too-tight jeans).

Of course, everyone responds differently to training. In addition to how hard and how consistently you exercise (and how well you manage your caloric intake), your results will also be determined by genetics. You can't change the unique genetic design that gives you an apple- or pear-shaped body, or a slight, medium, or heavy build, but you can look better than you ever have. Strength training balances out your body shape, helping you camouflage "problem" areas.

As you get stronger, slimmer, and more toned, you'll be healthier, leaner, more energetic, and more confident. You'll simply feel good about being in your body.

START NOW

All you have to do is turn the page to begin your first mini-workout. Have fun!

8 | Workout One: Strength and Stability

BUILDING YOUR BASE

The first step in lower-body training is restoring functional strength, mobility, and coordination to your leg and buttock muscles. When your legs are strong enough to support your body weight, you can safely and efficiently perform all of your daily activities, from loading your car with heavy grocery bags to running a few miles after work.

ABOUT THE EXERCISES

In Workout One, you'll be using your body weight as resistance. Practicing these compound exercises works both major and supporting muscles, strengthening your lower body, improving your balance, increasing your hip and knee joint mobility, improving your posture and torso stability, working your abdominal muscles, and improving your muscle tone.

The exercises may look simple, but if you practice them in correct form, making slow, controlled movements, you'll feel your quads, hamstrings, and glutes start to burn as you reach the end of your reps. Stretching after each exercise, or after your workout, will improve your muscle flexibility, range of motion, and overall strength. Don't be surprised if you're sore the next day. These moves really burn your butt.

If you find it difficult to perform the suggested number of reps, just do as many as you can. With time, you'll work up to more. Once you master each exercise, then you can try some of the modifications as long as you can maintain correct form while performing them.

BEFORE YOU BEGIN

If you haven't already read chapters 1 through 7, please do so before practicing any of the exercises in this book. These chapters contain essential training techniques, exercise guidelines, and safety information that are vital to your success. Most important, remember the description of correct posture on page 51 (chest up, shoulders down, etc.).

After reading this chapter, read all of the exercise instructions at least one more time to familiarize yourself with the different movements, breathing techniques, and postural tips you'll use during each exercise. The more prepared you are, the more successful you'll be.

Remember, you'll need to warm up for five to ten minutes before practicing each workout and cool down for the same amount of time afterward. After six to eight weeks, progress to Workout Two.

EXERCISE 1: THE SQUAT

In a survey of **36,000** American Council on Exercise–certified personal trainers (ACE), the squat was rated the most effective exercise for strengthening and toning the thighs and glutes. It's also an excellent functional exercise; you perform a squat every time you sit down.

Targets: quads, hamstrings, glutes, abductors, adductors, lower back, abs

Starting Position

Stand tall in correct posture, with feet hips-width apart and arms extended in front of you, parallel to each other and to the floor. Pull abs up and in toward spine.

Action

1. As if you were sitting down in a chair, inhale as you lower your body until your thighs are parallel to the floor, reaching behind you with your butt and bending slightly forward at the

hips. Sink your weight into your heels. Keep your chest up, back straight, eyes looking straight ahead.

Figure 8.1 *Squat*

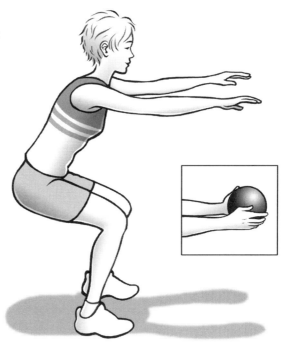

2. Pause for 1 to 2 seconds. Imagine that someone is gently pulling your fingertips forward and another person is behind you, gently pulling your hips behind you. Exhale as you slowly return to starting position by pushing off against the floor with your feet. Do 1 to 3 sets of 8 to 10 reps.

Technique Tips

- Maintain abs-to-spine, neutral spine, and correct posture throughout exercise. Keep heels in contact with the floor.
- Use leg and glute muscles to initiate movement, not back muscles.
- Don't allow knees to extend past toes. It's okay if you can't lower your body all the way to the "thighs parallel with floor" position, just don't go past parallel.
- Don't forget to breathe during pause.

Modifications

- Increase intensity by (1) starting with arms at sides, raising them and reaching forward as you squat, or (2) squatting while holding dumbbells to your chest, wearing a weighted vest, or holding a medicine ball in front of you. *(See Figure 8.1 inset.)*

- Decrease intensity by squatting in front of your bed. Lower your body until your butt touches the bed, then return to starting position. Or, squat behind a chair so that you can place your hands on the back of the chair for stability.

You'll Feel It: in your quads and hamstrings as you lower your body and in your glutes when you raise your body.

EXERCISE 2: LUNGE

ACE-certified personal trainers rated the lunge a very close second to the squat for strengthening and shaping the glutes. This functional exercise helps prepare you for such activities as climbing stairs and picking up objects from the floor. The lunge challenges your balance, so it might take a bit of practice to get it right.

Targets: quads, hamstrings, glutes, calves, lower back, abs

Starting Position

Stand tall in correct posture, feet 6 inches to hips-width apart. Pull abs up and in toward spine.

Action

1. Inhale as you lower yourself into the lunge position, taking a large step forward with your left foot and dropping your weight into your back leg as you bend your right knee toward the floor. Your right heel will come off the floor but your right knee should not touch the floor.

   As you lower your torso, bend slightly forward at the hips, raising your right arm forward until your upper arm is approaching parallel with the floor, and move your left arm backward until your forearm is approaching perpendicular with the floor (i.e., use the same arm motion as you do when running). (*See Figure 8.2.*)
2. Pause for 1 to 2 seconds. Exhale as you push off with your left foot to return to starting position. Do 1 to 3 sets of 8 to 10 reps for each leg.

feel in back leg.

Technique Tips

• Maintain abs-to-spine, neutral spine, and correct posture throughout exercise.

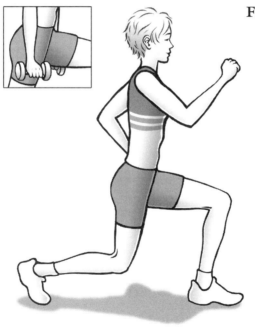

Figure 8.2 *Lunge*

- Keep hips squared and facing forward.
- Don't lean as far forward as you did in the squat.
- Remember, your goal isn't moving forward, but dropping your torso straight toward the floor.
- Don't lower your body past "thighs parallel to the floor," don't extend knee of front leg past toes, and don't allow knee of back leg to touch the floor.
- Return to starting position by pushing off with front foot; do not initiate movement with your back muscles.
- Keep arms and legs bent at (approximately) 90 degrees.

Modifications

- Increase intensity by lunging while holding dumbbells (arms at sides), wearing a weighted vest, or holding a medicine ball (at chest level). *(See Figure 8.2 inset.)*
- Decrease intensity by practicing lunge with hands on hips to aid balance or by lunging next to a chair for support.

You'll Feel It: in your quads, hamstrings, and glutes.

EXERCISE 3:
BENT KNEE CROSSOVER WITH LEG EXTENSION

This hip-firming exercise improves strength, stability, and range of motion in the hip joints.

Targets: glutes, hamstrings, abductors, adductors

Starting Position

Kneel on all fours, hands aligned under shoulders, knees aligned under hips. Pull abs up and in toward spine.

Action

1. Keeping your right leg bent at a 90-degree angle, slowly lift it until your thigh is lined up behind your right buttock and parallel to the floor. *(See Figure 8.3a.)*
2. Keeping your right leg bent at a 90-degree angle, slowly lower your right knee to the outside of your left leg. (It's

okay if you can't touch the floor with your right knee.) *(See Figure 8.3b.)*

3. Slowly raise your right leg back across your left leg until your thigh is parallel to the floor and extended behind your right buttock. Then straighten your right leg behind you, keeping it parallel to the floor. Pause for 1 to 2 seconds, then return to starting position. *(See Figure 8.3c.)* Do 1 to 3 sets of 8 to 10 reps on each leg.

Figure 8.3

Bent Knee Crossover with Leg Extension

8.3a

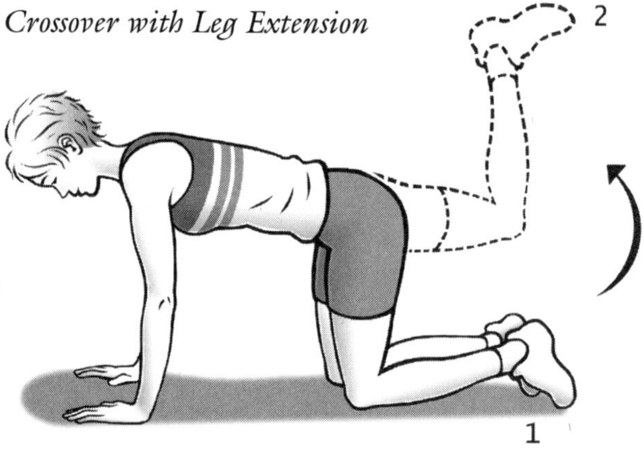

Workout One: Strength and Stability

8.3b

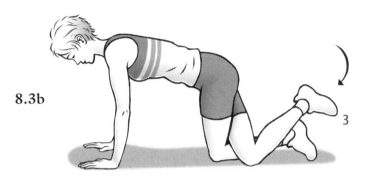

3

8.3c

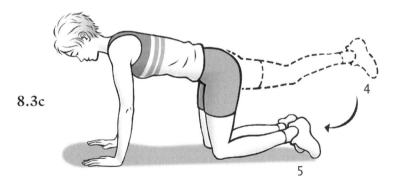

4

5

Technique Tips

- Maintain abs-to-spine, neutral spine, and correct posture throughout exercise.
- Squeeze together buttocks to keep glutes active. Don't arch your lower back.
- Keep hips squared and facing the floor. Imagine that there's a plate of loose grapes sitting on the back of your hips; to prevent the grapes from falling off the plate, don't allow one side of your hips to raise with movement.
- Keep both legs bent at 90 degrees.
- Breathe normally, and don't forget to breathe during pause.

Modifications

- Increase intensity by wearing 1- to 2-pound ankle weights on active leg.
- Decrease intensity by eliminating step 2 (extending active leg).

You'll Feel It: in your hips, outer thighs, and glutes.

EXERCISE 4:
FIRE HYDRANT WITH
LEG EXTENSION

Like the previous exercise, the fire hydrant gives you firm, functional hips.

Targets: glutes, hamstrings, abductors, adductors

Starting Position

Kneel on all fours, hands aligned under shoulders, knees aligned under hips. Pull abs up and in toward spine. *(See Figure 8.4a.)*

Action

1. Keeping your right leg bent at a 90-degree angle, slowly lift it up and away from the right side of your body. (If you've ever seen a dog utilize a fire hydrant, you know this movement.) Stop raising your right leg before you feel like raising your right hip. Pause for 1 to 2 seconds. *(See Figure 8.4b.)*

2. Slowly lower your right leg to starting position, then extend and straighten it behind you, keeping it parallel to the floor. Pause for 1 to 2 seconds. *(See Figure 8.4c.)*
3. Slowly return to starting position. Do 1 to 3 sets of 8 to 10 reps on each leg.

Technique Tips

• Maintain abs-to-spine, neutral spine, and correct posture throughout exercise. Don't arch your back.

Figure 8.4
Fire Hydrant with Leg Extension

8.4a

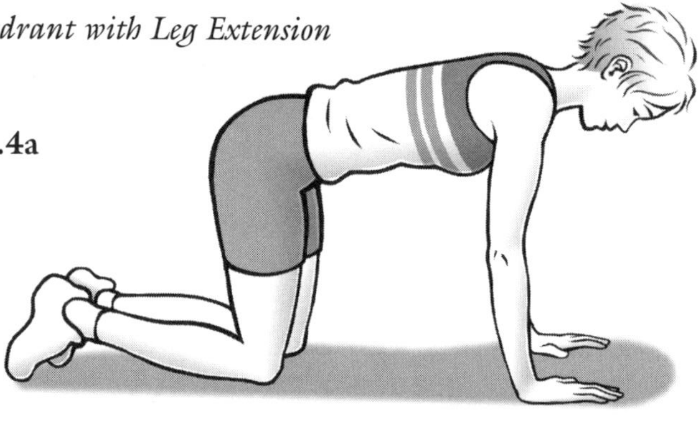

Workout One: Strength and Stability

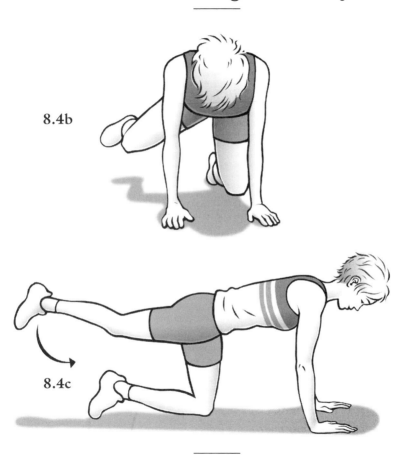

8.4b

8.4c

- Keep hips squared and facing the floor. Don't allow one side of your hips to raise with movement.
- Keep both legs bent at 90 degrees.
- Breathe normally, and don't forget to breathe during pause.

Modifications

- Increase intensity by wearing a 1- to 2-pound ankle weight on active leg.
- Decrease intensity by eliminating step 2 (extending active leg).

You'll Feel It: in your hips, inner thighs, and glutes.

9 | Workout Two: Wide-Leg Moves

SLIMMER HIPS AND THIGHS

If you hike, dance, play sports, or if you've ever had to jump onto the curb to avoid oncoming traffic, you know that the path from A to B is rarely a straight line. Your legs need to be strong enough to shuffle, sidestep, crouch, and jump in all directions. Strengthening your hips and inner thighs will improve your stability during lateral movements and help get your thighs and bum bikini ready.

ABOUT THE EXERCISES

All of the exercises in Workout Two are adaptations of common exercises and movements that challenge your muscles in a variety of positions to help you build and maintain lower-body strength.

You may not see the difference between the lunge and the squat in this workout and in Workout One. They do look very similar, and they both strengthen the same muscles. However, by changing the stance of the squat and the direction of the lunge (in this workout), you'll feel the burn more in your inner thighs, glutes, and hips.

The bridge exercise will challenge you to recruit the right muscles for the job (primarily, the glutes) while maintaining correct posture and pelvic alignment. You should only progress to the bridge modification if you have mastered correct form. Finally, the band walk is a fun, simple exercise that you'll feel in your glutes and hips.

Workout Two: Wide-Leg Moves

EQUIPMENT NEEDED

You'll need a resistance band (a paper-thin, flat ribbon of rubber about four inches wide and four feet long) or tubing (a rubber tube about a centimeter thick and four feet long) for the bridge and band walk exercises. Bands and tubing come in a variety of resistance levels, signified by color. Make sure you get a band that provides enough resistance. You can buy bands and tubing by the roll (split a roll with friends for a very inexpensive supply) or precut, usually to four feet, for about $3 or $4.

You can use the same piece of band or tubing in the band walk if it provides enough resistance; just tie it in a knot to make a loop. Or, you can buy premade loops. A basic band loop costs about the same as a band, and a tubing loop, which usually has foam pads on each side of the loop where it rests against your legs, costs about $8 to $12. You might want to buy two bands that provide different levels of resistance so that when you're ready to increase your resistance, you have the appropriate equipment.

(See page 163, Resources, for a list of exercise band and tubing manufacturers.)

EXERCISE 1: WIDE STANCE SQUAT

Widening your stance in this squat variation really works your inner thighs, helping you firm up the flab.

Targets: quads, hamstrings, glutes, abductors, adductors, lower back, abs

Starting Position

Stand tall in correct posture, with feet quite a bit more than hips-width apart in a wide stance, arms extended in front of you, parallel to each other and the floor. Rotate feet slightly outward (about 10 degrees). Pull abs up and in toward spine.

Action

1. As if you were sitting down in a chair, inhale as you lower your torso toward the floor until your thighs are parallel to the floor, reaching behind you with your butt, and bending slightly forward at the hips. Sink your weight into your heels.

Workout Two: Wide-Leg Moves

Keep your chest up, back straight, eyes looking straight ahead.

Figure 9.1
Wide Stance Squat

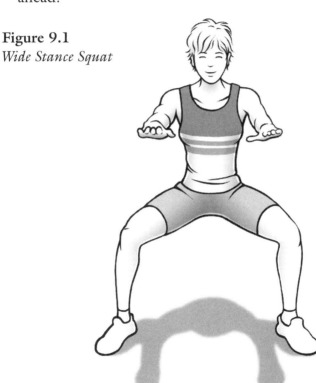

2. Pause for 1 to 2 seconds. Imagine that someone is gently pulling your fingertips forward and another person is behind you, gently pulling your hips behind you. Exhale as you slowly return to starting position by pushing off against the floor with your feet. Do 1 to 3 sets of 8 to 10 reps.

Technique Tips

- Maintain abs-to-spine, neutral spine, and correct posture throughout exercise.
- Use legs and glutes to initiate movement, not back muscles.
- You'll notice that you won't be able to lean as far forward as you did in the regular squat.
- Don't allow knees to extend past toes, and don't lower your body past the "thighs parallel to the floor" point.
- Don't forget to breathe during the pause.

Modifications

- Increase intensity by (1) starting with arms at sides, raising them and reaching forward as you squat, or (2) squatting while holding dumbbell (to your chest), wearing a weighted vest, or holding a medicine ball (arms extended in front of you).

- Decrease intensity by squatting in front of a chair. Lower your body until your butt touches the chair, then return to starting position. Or, squat behind a chair so that you can place your hands on the chair back for stability.

You'll Feel It: in your quads, glutes, and inner thighs.

EXERCISE 2: SIDE LUNGE

Side lunges give you sleek, strong thighs, firm up your bum, and improve lower-body strength, balance, and flexibility. You'll need to be patient with this one; it takes a while to master correct form.

Targets: quads, hamstrings, glutes, abductors, adductors, lower back, abs

Starting Position

Stand tall in correct posture, with feet hips-width apart, arms extended in front of you, parallel to each other and to the floor. Pull abs up and in toward spine.

Action

1. Inhale as you take a large step to the left with your left foot, lowering your body into the lunge position by bending your left knee and sitting into your left heel. As you lower your body, bend forward very slightly at the hips. Reach behind you with your butt as if you'll be sitting on a chair when you reach the side lunge position. Keep your hips squared, and

align your left knee over your left ankle. Your right leg should remain straight, with knee slightly bent.

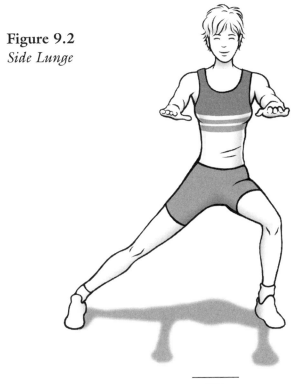

Figure 9.2
Side Lunge

2. Pause for 1 to 2 seconds. Exhale, pressing off with your left foot to return to starting position. Do 1 to 3 sets of 8 to 10 reps on each leg.

Technique Tips

- Maintain abs-to-spine, neutral spine, and correct posture throughout exercise. Keep your chest up.
- Make sure that your hips are squared and facing forward, feet parallel.
- Step out far enough to the side to correctly align your knee over your ankle, but not so far that you strain any muscles or compromise form. Don't allow the knee of your bent leg to extend past your toes.
- If your heels come off the floor, your stance is too wide.
- Initiate movement with your leg and glute muscles, not your back muscles.

Modifications

- Increase intensity by (1) starting with arms at sides, raising them into extended, reaching position as you lower yourself into the lunge; or (2) lunging while holding dumbbells (arms at sides), wearing a weighted vest, or holding a medicine ball (arms extended).

- Decrease intensity by (1) starting in a wide-leg stance so that you can lower yourself into the lunge position without taking a step or (2) placing a chair behind you at the end of the lunge and touching your butt to it.

You'll Feel It: in your quads, hamstrings, glutes, adductors, and abductors.

EXERCISE 3: BRIDGE

This yoga-inspired exercise is great for tightening and toning the glutes.

Targets: hamstrings and glutes

Figure 9.3
Bridge

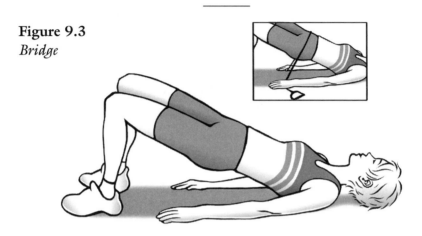

Starting Position

Lie on your back with your knees bent, heels about 9 to 12 inches in front of buttocks, arms at sides. Pull abs up and in toward spine. Squeeze together buttocks. Inhale.

Action

1. Exhale, raising your pelvis toward the ceiling until your knees, hips, and shoulders form a straight line. Your shoulder

blades should maintain contact with the floor. *(See Figure 9.3.)*

2. Pause for 1 to 2 seconds. Exhale, slowly lowering your pelvis to the floor. Do 1 to 3 sets of 8 to 10 reps.

Technique Tips

• Maintain abs-to-spine, neutral spine, and correct posture throughout exercise. Squeeze buttocks to protect lower back. Press into floor with feet for stability.
• Use glutes to initiate movement, not your back muscles.

Modification

• Increase intensity by keeping arms at sides and holding a rubber fitness band or tube across the front of the pelvis to make lifting the pelvis more challenging. *(See Figure 9.3 inset.)*

You'll Feel It: in your glutes and your hamstrings. (You should not feel it in your lower back.)

EXERCISE 4:
MINI-BAND SHUFFLE

This fun exercise, also called the Monster Walk, is a deceptively simple way to get legs of steel.

Targets: quads, hamstrings, glutes, abductors, adductors, lower back, abs

Starting Position

Stand tall in correct posture, arms at sides, feet 6 to 8 inches greater than hips-width apart with a rubber tube or band around both legs, just above the ankles. Stance should be wide enough to make the band taut. Pull abs up and in toward spine.

Action

1. Maintaining constant tension against the band, and keeping feet parallel, slowly walk forward (using small, shuffling steps) for 20 to 40 steps. *(See Figure 9.4.)*

2. Shuffle backward the same amount of steps. Repeat sequence 8 to 10 times.

Technique Tips

• Maintain correct posture, with chest up, hips squared and facing forward, and eyes looking straight ahead. Keep your abs engaged to maintain neutral spine. Don't use your back muscles to initiate movement.

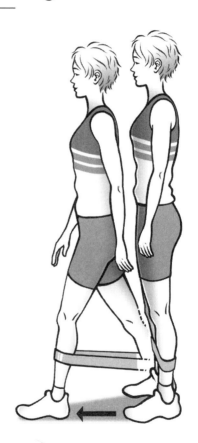

Figure 9.4
Mini-Band Shuffle

- Make sure that you use a band with enough resistance to challenge your lower-body muscles.
- Keep knees aligned over first and second toes; use your glutes to prevent your knees from caving in toward each other.
- In order to maintain band tension on legs, take small, shuffle steps rather than rolling feet from heel to toe with each step.

Modification

- Increase intensity by bending knees (until you're in a one-quarter squat), then walking; or by using a band that provides greater resistance.

You'll Feel It: in your thighs and glutes.

10 | Workout Three: One-Legged Moves

CHALLENGING BALANCE

Most people don't think about their balance until they feel unsteady walking up a flight of stairs or balancing on one leg to pick up something from the floor. Practicing exercises that challenge your balance engages all your lower-body muscles in supporting and controlling your body weight. The one-legged moves in this workout will improve your strength and balance *and* give you firm, defined thighs and a rock-hard butt.

ABOUT THE EXERCISES

In Workout Three, you'll be increasing the difficulty of exercises similar to those in Workouts One and Two by balancing on one leg while working the other leg. (In most of the exercises, your balancing leg will get quite a workout, too!)

Balancing exercises are effective at building integrated strength because they challenge muscles, connective tissues, nerves, and joints to work together to support the body. As you practice each exercise, you'll be retraining your muscles and reprogramming your nervous system to adapt to each movement. With time, you'll establish new, healthy movement patterns so that you'll move with more strength, grace, and coordination.

Now that you're adding balance work to your routine, correct form is even more important. Always use your abs to protect your lower back.

Equipment Needed

In Exercise 2, you'll need to use the bottom step of a staircase. Or, if you have aerobics steps, you can use those instead. I prefer aerobics steps because I can begin with a height of only four to six inches, gradually increasing the height as I improve.

You'll need an exercise band or tubing for Exercise 4. Read the "Equipment Needed" section on page 89 for more information on bands and tubing.

EXERCISE 1:
SINGLE LEG SQUAT ON STEP

Single leg squats really turn up the heat on lower-body muscles, improving balance, strength, and muscle definition.

Targets: quads, hamstrings, glutes, abductors, adductors, lower back, abs

Starting Position

Stand tall in correct posture on the bottom step of a staircase (or better, on the edge of an aerobics step that's 12 to 15 inches high), left side facing the stairs. Extend arms in front of your body, parallel to each other and to the floor. Pull abs up and in toward spine.

Action

1. As if you were sitting down in a chair, inhale as you slowly lower your body, reaching behind you with your butt and bending slightly forward at the hips. Drop your weight into your left heel. Keep your right leg straight, toes flexed, so that only your heel briefly makes contact with the floor (below the step) when you lower your body into the squat. (This prevents you from using the right leg to balance yourself or push off with.) If you're using a high step, you won't be able to touch the floor with your heel. *(See Figure 10.1.)*

2. Pause for 1 to 2 seconds. Exhale, pushing into the step with your left foot to return to starting position. Do 1 to 3 sets of 8 to 10 reps on each leg.

Figure 10.1
Single Leg Squat on Step

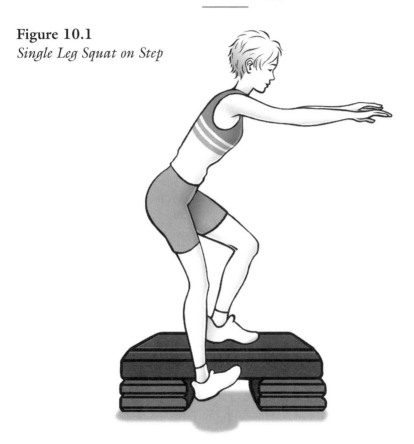

Technique Tips

- Maintain abs-to-spine, neutral spine, and correct posture throughout exercise.
- You'll notice that you won't be able to bend as far forward at the hips as you would during a traditional squat. Keep your chest up, eyes looking straight ahead.
- You probably won't be able to lower your body until your left thigh is parallel with the floor—most people can't.
- Visualize that someone is in front of you, gently pulling on your fingertips, and another person is behind you, gently pulling your hips behind you.
- Keep hips squared (don't let one hip hike up with movement), and don't allow your bent knee to extend past your toes.

Modification

- Increase intensity by using a higher step, holding weights (at sides or at chest) or a medicine ball (at chest or with extended arms), or wearing a weighted vest.

You'll Feel It: in your quads, hamstrings, and glutes.

EXERCISE 2:
LUNGE WITH RAISED BACK LEG

This move is also called a split squat. It's another excellent functional exercise for improving balance and flexibility and building integrated strength.

Targets: quads, hamstrings, glutes, abductors, adductors, lower back, abs

Starting Position

Stand in correct posture, arms extended in front of you, with your back to a staircase or small stool (approximately 8 to 12 inches high), calves touching the front of the lowest step. Pull abs up and in toward spine. Take a large step forward with your left foot, then place your right foot on the top of the stair (toes flexed against the surface).

Action

1. Inhale as you lower your torso into the lunge position, bending both knees and sitting into your back leg. Bend forward at the hips very slightly, keeping your chest up, back straight, and both knees bent at (approximately) 90-degree angles. Your right heel will come off the step. *(See Figure 10.2.)*
2. Pause for 1 to 2 seconds. Exhale as you push off with your left foot to return to starting position. Do 1 to 3 sets of 8 to 10 reps for each leg.

Technique Tips

- Maintain abs-to-spine, neutral spine, and correct posture throughout exercise.
- You'll notice that you won't be able to lean forward as much as you do in a squat or in a regular lunge.
- Keep your hips squared and facing forward.
- Do not lower your body past the "thigh parallel to the floor" point.
- Keep knee of front leg in line with first and second toes; do not extend knee of front leg past toes or allow it to cave in.

Workout Three: One-Legged Moves

Figure 10.2
*Lunge with Raised
Back Leg*

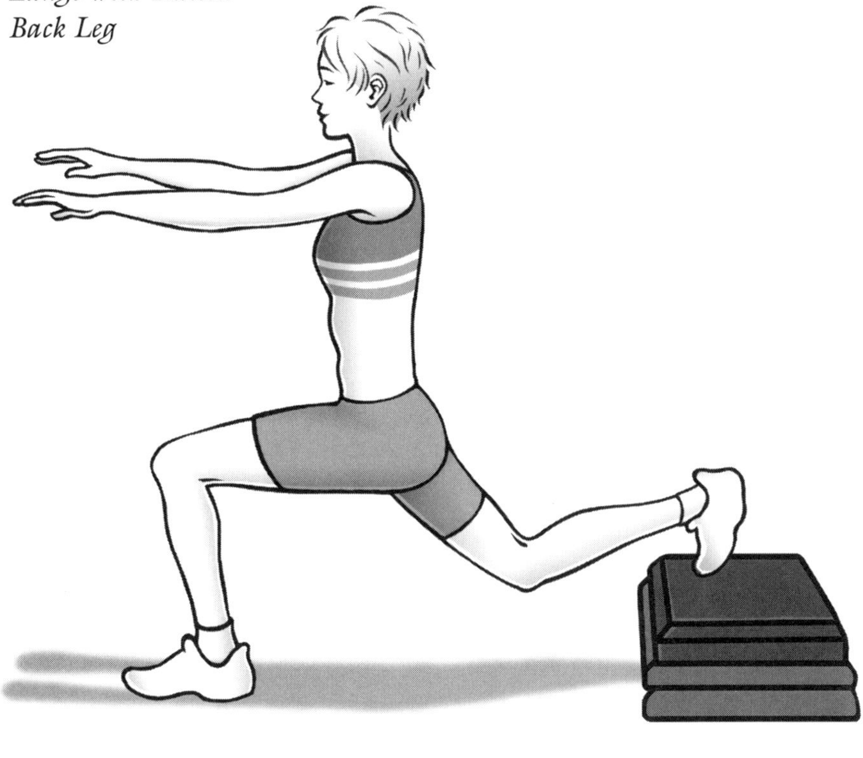

Modifications

- Increase intensity by (1) starting with arms at sides, extending them and reaching forward with fingertips at the same time you squat; (2) holding dumbbells (arms at sides), wearing a weighted vest, or holding a medicine ball (at chest or arms extended); (3) raising the height of the step to 15 inches, then to chair height; or (4) replace step with stability ball (after receiving instruction from physical therapist or certified personal trainer).
- Decrease intensity by using a lower step (6 to 8 inches high).

You'll Feel It: in your quads, hamstrings, and glutes.

EXERCISE 3:
ONE-LEGGED BRIDGE

This butt-blasting move will firm you up fast. It's also easy to include in a Pilates or yoga routine since you're already on the floor.

Targets: glutes, hamstrings

Starting Position

Lie on your back with your knees bent, heels about 6 to 12 inches in front of buttocks, arms at sides, palms down. (*See Figure 10.3a.*) Pull abs up and in toward spine. Raise right knee toward chest, and let it rest there. Squeeze together buttocks. Inhale.

Action

1. Keeping right leg raised and relaxed, exhale as you slowly raise your pelvis toward the ceiling until your left knee, hip, and shoulder form a straight line. Shoulder blades should maintain contact with floor. (*See Figure 10.3b.*)

Figure 10.3
One-Legged Bridge

10.3a

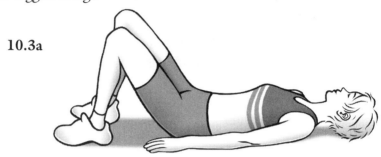

10.3b

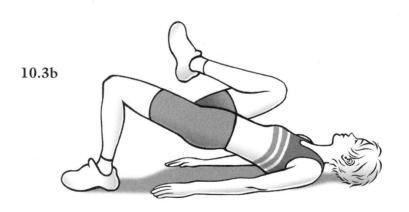

Workout Three: One-Legged Moves

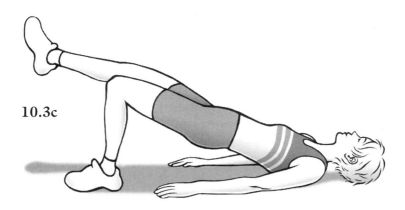

10.3c

2. Pause for 1 to 2 seconds. Inhale as you slowly lower your pelvis to the floor using your glutes (and keeping your back straight). Do 1 to 3 sets of 8 to 10 reps on each leg.

Technique Tips

• Maintain abs-to-spine, neutral spine, and correct posture throughout exercise. Maintain buttock squeeze to protect lower back. Press into floor with working foot for stability.

- Keep hips squared. Don't hike up one side of your hips.
- Initiate movement with glutes, not with lower-back muscles.

Modifications

- Increase the intensity by (1) placing arms at sides, palms up (to prevent you from pressing hands against floor) or bending arms at 90 degrees (so that only forearms are touching floor); or (2) performing one-legged bridge with right leg extended. *(See Figure 10.3c.)*

You'll Feel It: in your glutes and your hamstrings. (You should not feel it in your lower back.)

EXERCISE 4: FOUR-WAY HIP MOTION WITH BAND

Healthy joints are the key to maintaining your mobility. This exercise improves lower-body strength while improving joint strength, range of motion, and overall body alignment. The bonus: You'll be so busy with your working leg that you won't notice how hard your standing leg is working until you've completed the exercise.

Targets: quads, hamstrings, glutes, abductors, adductors, lower back, abs

Starting Position

Attach a rubber exercise tube or band around the leg of an immovable heavy table (or better, close the attachment piece or knot behind a door). Place the other end of the loop around your left leg, just above the ankle. Stand tall in correct posture with your back facing, and a few feet in front of, the table (or door), arms extended in front of you, parallel to each other and to the floor. There should be tension on the band. Pull abs up and in toward spine. Inhale.

Action

1. Exhale as you slowly lift your left leg in front of you until the band stops you or you reach the end of your range of motion

(i.e., the point just before you want to move your hips or spine to move your left leg further). Pause for 1 to 2 seconds. Inhale as you slowly return your left leg to starting position. Do 8 to 10 reps. *(See Figure 10.4a.)*

2. Turn 90 degrees counter-clockwise so that your left side faces the table/door. Repeat exercise in this position, pulling your left leg across the front of your right leg. Do 8 to 10 reps. *(See Figure 10.4b.)*

3. Turn 90 degrees counter-clockwise again so that you're facing the table/door. Repeat exercise in this position, pulling your leg behind you. Do 8 to 10 reps. *(See Figure 10.4c.)*

4. Turn 90 degrees counter-clockwise so that your right side faces the table/door. Repeat exercise in this position, pulling your left leg away from your body. Do 8 to 10 reps. Do 1 to 3 sets of series. *(See Figure 10.4d.)*

Technique Tips

• Maintain abs-to-spine, neutral spine, and correct posture throughout exercise. Don't allow the hip of your moving leg to hike up with movement.

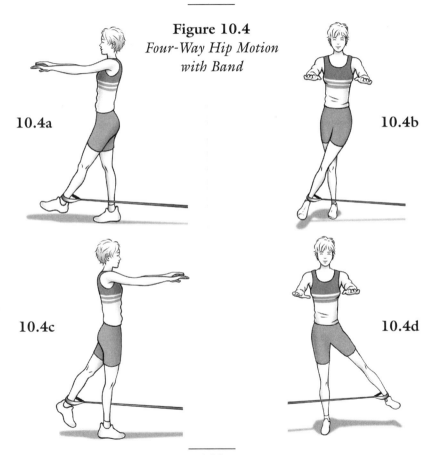

Figure 10.4
*Four-Way Hip Motion
with Band*

10.4a

10.4b

10.4c

10.4d

- Initiate movement with leg and glute muscles, not with lower back muscles. Don't use your spine or hips to move your leg.
- Keep legs straight, but not locked.
- Each time you change position, make sure that there is adequate tension on the band before you lift your leg.
- Use slow, controlled movements when lifting and lowering leg; do not rely on momentum.
- Make sure you use a band or tubing that provides enough resistance to make these movements challenging.

Modifications

- Increase intensity by using a band that provides greater resistance.
- Decrease intensity by practicing front, back, side, and crossover extensions without a band.

You'll Feel It: in your glutes, adductors, abductors, and in your standing leg.

11 | Workout Four: Killer Legs and Buns

THE FINAL CHALLENGE

Now that you have a strong base, you're ready for a killer workout that will challenge your strength and balance during movement, integrating lower-body and torso strength. These exercises will prepare you for such daily activities as reaching for and lifting weighted objects when squatting or in a crouching position and for the many movements you'll make playing sports. They'll also fine-tune your thighs, hips, and bum, giving your lower body that firm, cut look.

About These Exercises

Like the previous workouts, Workout Four contains exercises that will strengthen and shape your lower body and improve your coordination and balance. In addition, this workout provides the added benefit of strengthening core muscles (in the back and abdomen) and training lower-body and core muscles to work together to stabilize and support the spine during movement.

Protecting your lower back from injury by maintaining correct posture is critical—and much more difficult in these challenging exercises. Take your time learning correct form, and as always, pull your abs up and in toward your spine before movement.

Equipment Needed

You'll need a stability ball* (also called a balance ball or an exercise ball) for the Bridge on Ball exercise. (You can also use a chair or the edge of a sofa.) You can find balls at many sports stores and online fitness retailers for between $15 and $30. Balls come in a variety of sizes; make sure you buy the right ball for your height. In general, the following list of ball sizes and heights should help you select the right ball, but check with each manufacturer to confirm that their stability balls are sized according to the same heights.

- 45 cm ball (up to 4 ft. 10 in. tall)
- 55 cm ball (4 ft. 8 in. to 5 ft. 5 in.)
- 65 cm ball (5 ft. 5 in. to 6 ft. 0 in.)
- 75 cm ball (6 ft. 0 in. to 6 ft. 5 in.)
- 85 cm ball (6 ft. 5 in. or taller)

For your own safety, invest in a top-quality ball that is durable enough to support your body weight. Some of the

---

* Stability balls are excellent tools for strength, balance, and core training. If you'd like to learn more about stability ball exercises, read *The Little Abs Workout Book*.

less-expensive balls are no bargain: They're not as sturdy and they don't hold air as long as the better brands used by physical therapists and health clubs. A good ball should last for years. Some manufacturers make extra strong balls for use with dumbbells or other weights. See Resources for several ball manufacturers known for their quality products.

You'll also need a small 1- to 2-pound item for the lunge with reach exercise. You can use a dumbbell, a small medicine ball, a small bottle of water, or even a shoe.

EXERCISE 1: AIRPLANE AND ONE-LEGGED REACH

The airplane is another yoga-inspired exercise that improves balance, strengthens lower-body and back muscles, and improves hamstring and joint flexibility. Adding a reach to it (often called the "golfer's reach") further challenges balance. It's an effective functional exercise that builds integrated strength throughout the body and tones abdominal and lower-body muscles.

Targets: quads, hamstrings, glutes, abductors, adductors, lower back, abs

Starting Position

Stand tall in correct posture, feet hips-width apart, arms extended vertically over shoulders. Pull abs up and in toward spine. Inhale.

Action

1. Exhale as you bend forward at the hips, balancing on your left leg, until your body is parallel with the floor. Keep your right leg and arms in line with your torso, chest up, back and neck straight. Also, keep your hips squared, facing the floor. Point the toes of your right foot toward your right shin.

   Visualize that someone is standing in front of you, gently pulling on your fingers, and another person is standing behind you, gently pulling on your right heel to lengthen your spine. Pause for 1 to 2 seconds. Inhale as you raise yourself back to the starting position. Do 8 to 10 reps. *(See Figure 11.1, position 1.)*

Figure 11.1
Airplane

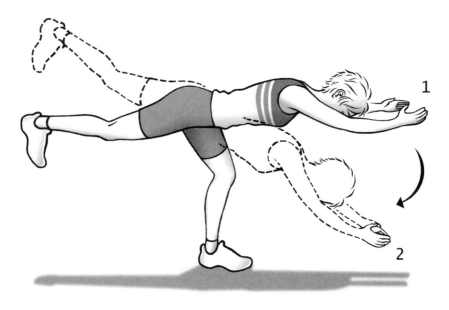

2. Once you can maintain your balance during the airplane, you can include the reach, position 2 (represented on Figure 11.1 by dotted lines). From the airplane position, pause for 1 to 2 seconds. Exhale as you slowly bend forward at the hips 45 to 60 degrees until you can touch the floor with your fingertips. Keep your right leg, arms, and torso straight and in line. Pause for 1 to 2 seconds. Inhale as you slowly raise yourself back to the starting position. Do 8 to 10 reps. Do 1 to 3 sets of this series.

Technique Tips

- Maintain abs-to-spine, neutral spine, and correct posture throughout exercise.
- Don't forget to use your abs when returning to starting position.
- Focus on your breathing during the pauses to help you maintain your balance and protect your lower back.
- Keep hips squared, as if you're balancing a plate of loose grapes on your lower back.
- Understand that it's okay to bend your standing leg if necessary.

Modifications

- Increase intensity by holding a 1-pound medicine ball (arms extended).
- Decrease intensity by bending forward only 45 degrees, then 60 degrees, and working up to 90 degrees in step 1. You can also hold your arms in a "T" position to aid in balance.

You'll Feel It: in your legs, hips, and lower back.

EXERCISE 2: LUNGE WITH REACH

Every day you reach for several objects at different heights and at different distances from your body. This lunge variation helps improve strength, balance, and coordination, preparing you for such movements as stepping closer to a table to reach your car keys and lowering your body to reach for a suitcase.

Targets: quads, hamstrings, glutes, abductors, adductors, lower back, abs

Starting Position

Place a shoe on the edge of a table. Stand tall in correct posture about 3 to 4 feet in front of the table. Feet should be 6 inches to hips-width apart, arms extended in front of you. Pull abs up and in toward spine.

Action

1. Inhale as you lower your torso straight toward the floor by taking a large step forward with your left foot and dropping your weight into your back leg as you bend your right knee toward the floor. Your right heel will come off the floor, but your right knee should not touch the floor. Both of your legs should form (approximately) 90-degree angles. As you lower your torso, bend slightly forward at the hips so that your torso lines up with your right thigh. Once in the lunge position, pick up the shoe, and pull it to your chest. *(See Figure 11.2a.)*
2. Pause for 1 to 2 seconds. Exhale as you push off with your left foot to return to the starting position. Do 1 to 3 sets of 8 to 10 reps for each leg.

Figure 11.2
Lunge with Reach

11.2a

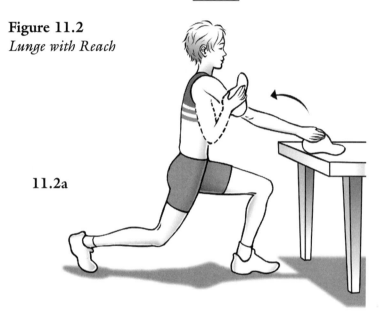

3. Next, practice the lunge and reach in front of a chair. To reach lower, inhale as you go a bit deeper into the lunge while keeping your legs bent at approximately 90 degrees. You may bend slightly forward at the hips, keeping back straight, to reach shoe with hands. Once you reach the shoe, pull it to your chest. Pause 1 to 2 seconds. Exhale as you

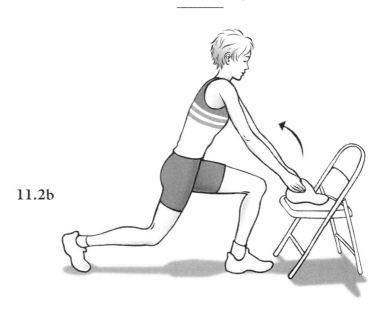

11.2b

    push off with your left foot to return to the starting position. Do 8 to 10 reps. *(See Figure 11.2b.)*

4. If you've mastered steps 1 through 3, try lunging and reaching for an object on the floor. You may have to bend forward at the hips a bit to reach the shoe, but keep your back straight. Do 8 to 10 reps. *(See Figure 11.2c.)* You can

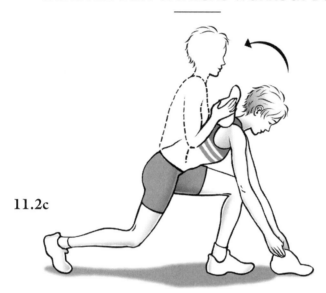

11.2c

do 1 to 3 sets of lunge with reach, or do all three lunges with reaches for a 3-set exercise.

Technique Tips

- Maintain abs-to-spine, neutral spine, and correct posture throughout exercise. Keep chest up when bending forward at the hips to maintain posture.

- Your goal isn't moving forward, but dropping your torso straight toward the floor.
- Make sure that your hips are squared and facing forward.
- Do not lower your body past thigh-parallel-to-floor position and do not extend knee of front leg past toes.
- Initiate your return to starting position by pressing off with your front foot, not by using back muscles.

Modifications

- Increase intensity by reaching for (and lifting) a small dumbbell or weighted ball (use 1 to 2 pounds at first, then increase resistance very gradually). Lift the item by pulling it straight to your chest. Then return to starting position. With your next lunge, begin with the weight at your chest, and when you reach, replace the item. Alternate reaching and lifting and returning the item with each lunge.
- Decrease intensity by reaching for, but not lifting, objects.

You'll Feel It: in your quads, hamstrings, and glutes.

EXERCISE 3: BRIDGE ON BALL

Bridging on a ball gives you more bang for your buck. As you work against instability and resistance, all your lower-body muscles have to work together to move your body, firming your backside and flattening your stomach.

Targets: hamstrings, glutes, lower back, abs

Starting Position

Lie on your back with your lower legs resting on a stability ball, ankles 3 to 4 inches to hips-width apart. Let your arms rest at your sides, palms down. Pull abs up and in toward spine. Squeeze together buttocks. Inhale. *(See Figure 11.3a.)*

Action

1. Exhale as you slowly raise your pelvis toward the ceiling, pressing your heels into the ball, until your ankles, knees, hips, and shoulders form a straight line. Your shoulder blades should maintain contact with the floor. *(See Figure 11.3b.)*

Workout Four: Killer Legs and Buns

Figure 11.3
Bridge on Ball

11.3a

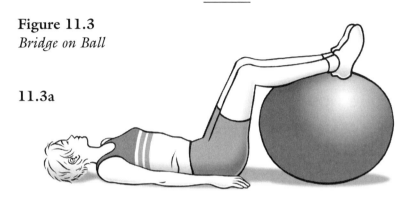

11.3b

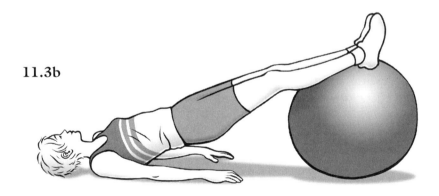

2. Pause for 1 to 2 seconds. Exhale as you slowly lower your pelvis to the floor using your glutes (and keeping your back straight). Do 1 to 3 sets of 8 to 10 reps.

Technique Tips

- Maintain abs-to-spine, neutral spine, and correct posture throughout exercise.
- Use slow, controlled movements.
- Don't press into the floor with your hands.
- Initiate movement with your glutes, not with lower-back muscles.

Modifications

- Increase intensity by practicing bridge: (1) with palms up, or (2) with one leg. Start with left leg bent at 90 degrees, left calf resting on the ball, right leg pulled toward chest in a relaxed position. Use glutes to raise pelvis into bridge position.
- Decrease intensity by moving ankles a bit wider apart in starting position.

You'll Feel It: in your glutes, hamstrings, and lower-back muscles.

EXERCISE 4:
SIDE LYING PLANK WITH LEG LIFT

You don't need a ball to create instability. This super-strengthening move really challenges your alignment, posture, and balance, helping you develop a toned tummy, firmer hips, and tighter thighs.

Targets: abs, abductors, adductors

Starting Position

Lie on your right side with your thighs together, right leg bent at approximately 90 degrees, left knee straight and in line with your torso, left hand on your hip. Pull abs up and in toward spine. Using your right forearm for support, raise your upper body until your right shoulder, hip, and knee line up, leaving your right hip in contact with the floor. (Your right arm should be bent at 90 degrees, elbow below shoulder, fingers facing away from your body.)

Action

1. Inhale as you slowly raise your left leg until it's parallel to the floor. Keep it straight, with toes pointed away from your body. *(See Figure 11.4a.)*
2. Pause for 1 to 2 seconds. Exhale as you lower your left leg. Do 1 to 3 sets of 8 to 10 reps on each leg.

Technique Tips

• Maintain abs-to-spine, neutral spine, and correct posture throughout exercise. Keep neck, back, and lifting leg in line. Raise chest, keep shoulders back, and push forearm (or hand) of working arm into the floor for support.

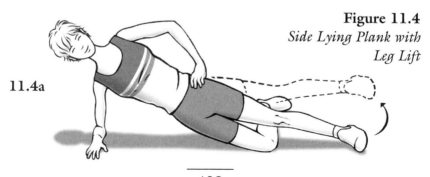

Figure 11.4
Side Lying Plank with Leg Lift

11.4a

Workout Four: Killer Legs and Buns

- Use slow, controlled movements to raise and lower active leg.
- Don't allow your right shoulder or your hips to roll forward. Keep your chest raised, pull your right shoulder back, and keep your hips squared.
- Use abdominal and lower-body muscles to initiate movement, not lower back muscles.

Modifications

- Increase intensity by (1) wearing ankle weights on working leg (start with 1- to 2-pound weights and gradually increase resistance) or (2) changing starting position by extending

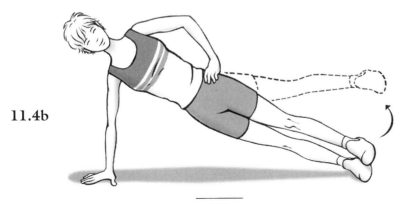

11.4b

supporting arm and bottom leg so that in the raised position, only your hand and the side of your foot are touching the floor. Then perform leg lift. *(See Figure 11.4b.)*

You'll Feel It: in your hips.

12 | Your Best Butt

ON YOUR WAY

With so many reshaping and resizing exercises from which to choose, plus a greater understanding of what your body needs to be healthy and functional, you're on your way to your best butt and bikini-ready thighs and hips.

STAY ON TRACK

The exercises in this book will keep you busy for months. Once you've mastered all four mini-workouts, you can mix and match exercises to create new workouts. I hope that you'll also be inspired to continue learning about exercise and its many benefits by reading additional information, attending fitness classes, or working with a fitness professional every now and then to fine-tune your workout. Exercising with a friend is another excellent way to stay motivated.

MAKE THE MOST OF EVERY MOVE

For best results: Every time you exercise, remember to pay attention to your form; use slow, controlled movements. And don't forget to *breathe!* The mini-workouts take only a few minutes, so please take your time and correctly practice each exercise so that you gain the most benefits.

NEW LIFESTYLE, NEW BODY

Just by eating a nutritious diet and exercising regularly, you'll be establishing healthy habits that will help you lose fat, gain muscle, and fit into your favorite clothes.

Your Best Butt

After two months, you'll have more energy, you'll feel strong and confident, and you'll look your best.

Good luck with reaching your fitness goals!

APPENDIX A
Lower-Body Stretches

STRONG AND SUPPLE

After practicing the exercises in this book, you'll have some tight muscles, so you need to spend at least five or ten minutes stretching. It's a good idea to consult a more thorough resource on lower-body stretching. However, to get you started, here are a few stretches to practice after each exercise or workout. Please use the illustrations to guide your position and movement.

APPENDIX A

STRETCHING TIPS

- Maintain neutral spine, correct posture, and alignment.
- Ease yourself into each stretch using slow, controlled movements.
- As you stretch, you'll feel tension in the muscle; do not push beyond that tension.
- Do not use jerky or bouncing movements.
- Relax your body, and continue breathing, inhaling and exhaling slowly and rhythmically.
- Try to go deeper into each stretch with inhalation, backing off a bit with each exhalation.
- Repeat each stretch a minimum of 4 to 8 times.
- When using a chair, place it against the wall to make it immovable.[1]

QUAD STRETCH

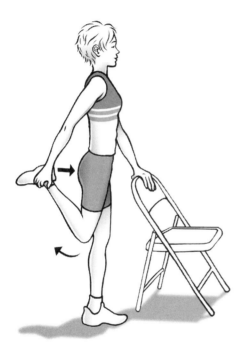

Figure A.1
Quad Stretch

Starting Position

Stand tall in correct posture, with your left hand resting on the back of a chair. Bend your right leg, raising your right heel toward your buttocks. Hold the top of your right foot (above the ankle) with your right hand. Keep thighs together. Squeeze the glutes of your bent leg. Inhale.

Action

1. Exhale as you slowly pull your right heel toward your right buttock and gently push your right hip

forward until you feel a stretch in your right thigh. Pause for 3 to 4 breaths (one breath = one inhalation + one exhalation). *(See Figure A.1.)*

2. Inhale as you release the stretch. Repeat with left leg.

HAMSTRING STRETCH

Starting Position

Stand tall in correct posture. Place the heel of your left foot on the seat of a chair (keeping left leg bent at about 120 degrees). Rest your hands just above the knee of your left leg. Pull toes of left foot toward shin. Inhale.

Lower-Body Stretches

Action

1. Exhale as you slowly straighten your left leg until you feel a stretch in your hamstring. Do not lock knees. Pause for 3 to 4 breaths. *(See Figure A.2.)*
2. Inhale as you raise your left knee. Repeat with right leg.

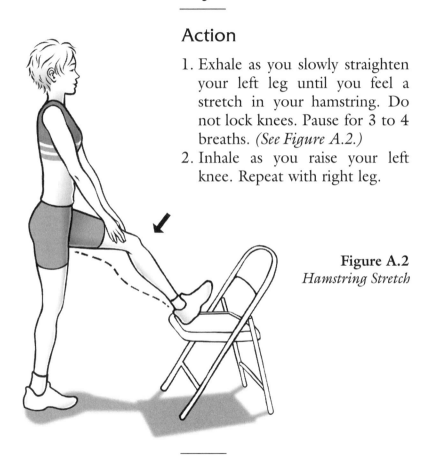

Figure A.2
Hamstring Stretch

HIP FLEXOR STRETCH

Starting Position

Stand tall in correct posture. Place left foot on the edge of a chair, slightly rotating toes of standing leg to the right, and rest hands on your thigh just above the knee. Squeeze glutes of standing leg. Inhale.

Action

1. Exhale as you slowly move your hips forward until you feel a stretch in the front of your hips (on right side). Pause for 3 to 4 breaths. Don't allow knee of raised leg to extend beyond toes. *(See Figure A.3.)*
2. Inhale as you return to starting position. Repeat with right leg.

Lower-Body Stretches

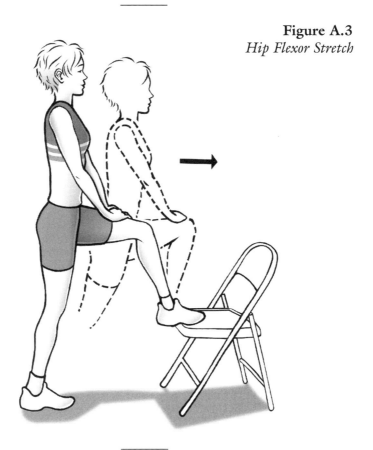

Figure A.3
Hip Flexor Stretch

BUTT STRETCH

Starting Position

Lie on your back, with your left leg bent at (approximately) 90 degrees. Bend your right leg, placing the outside of your ankle on your left thigh, just above the knee. Hold the back of your left thigh. Inhale.

Action

1. Exhale as you pull your left thigh toward your chest until you feel the stretch in your glutes. Pause in this position for 3 to 4 breaths. With each exhale, try to go a little bit deeper into the stretch. Release the stretch with an inhaling breath. *(See Figure A.4.)*
2. Repeat with right leg.

Figure A.4
Butt Stretch

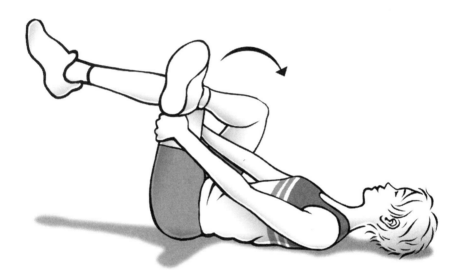

LOWER-BACK STRETCH

Starting Position

Lie on your back with your left leg bent, your left foot next to your right knee, and your arms extended from shoulders, perpendicular to your torso. Inhale.

Action

1. Exhale as you lower your left knee to (or toward) the floor, keeping your right leg straight and in line with your torso and your right hip touching the floor. Use your right hand to guide your left knee toward the floor and to keep it in stretched position. Pause for 6 to 8 breaths. You'll feel a stretch in your lower back and your left side lengthen as you breathe into your left side. Turn your head to the left to stretch your neck. *(See Figure A.5.)*
2. Inhale as you ease off the stretch. With each exhale, try to lower your right knee a little closer to the floor. Repeat with right leg.

Figure A.5
Lower-Back Stretch

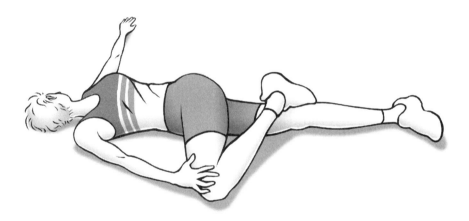

APPENDIX B
Calorie and Activity Charts

ESTIMATED CALORIE NEEDS FOR WOMEN AND MEN			
Weight (in pounds)	Daily activity level	Female calorie needs	Male calorie needs
130	Sedentary	1,716	1,888
130	Mildly active	1,859	2,045
130	Moderately active	2,002	2,202
130	Very active	2,145	2,360
140	Sedentary	1,848	2,033
140	Mildly active	2,002	2,202
140	Moderately active	2,156	2,372
140	Very active	2,310	2,541
150	Sedentary	1,980	2,178
150	Mildly active	2,145	2,360
150	Moderately active	2,310	2,541
150	Very active	2,475	2,743
160	Sedentary	2,112	2,323
160	Mildly active	2,288	2,517
160	Moderately active	2,464	2,710
160	Very active	2,640	2,904

APPENDIX B

ACTIVITY CALORIE-BURNING CHART

Activity (moderate intensity)	Duration	Calories burned (130-lb. person)	Calories burned (140-lb. person)	Calories burned (150-lb. person)	Calories burned (160-lb. person)
Aerobics (low impact)	30	172	185	198	211
Aerobics (high impact)	30	218	235	252	269
Bicycling (stationary)	30	218	235	252	269
Bicycling (outdoors)	30	312	336	360	384
Dancing (ballroom)	30	172	185	198	211
Elliptical trainer	30	281	302	324	346
Kayaking	30	156	168	180	192
Rowing machine	30	218	235	252	269
Strength training	30	94	101	108	115
Running	30	343	370	396	422
Walking	30	140	151	162	173
Yoga	30	125	134	144	154

Source: www.primusweb.com/fitnesspartner/, © 1995–2002 Fitness Jumpsite™ (Based on figures from the *Compendium of Physical Activity, ACSM's Resource Manual for Guidelines for Exercise Testing and Prescription,* 3rd ed. (Williams & Wilkins, 1998). Figures are approximate.

Notes

CHAPTER 2

1. Selene Yeager. "Banish Cellulite—In 20 Minutes!" *Prevention Magazine,* June 2001, page 150.

2. Wayne Westcott, Ph.D., Gary Reinl, and Donna Califano, PTA. "Strength Training for Older Adults." HealthWorld Online. www.healthy.net. 1998.

3. Wayne Westcott, Ph.D., CSCS, and Rita La Rosa Loud. *No More Cellulite.* Perigee (New York), 2003, page 12; Carol Krucoff. "Exercise for Bone Health." www.ivillage.health.com. 1998.

4. "How to Calculate Your Total Daily Calorie Needs." www.ehow.com; Kurt, Mike, and Brett Brundgardt. *The Complete Book of Butt and Legs.* Villard Books (New York), 1995, page 41.

5. Thomas R. Baechle and Roger W. Earle. *Essentials of Strength Training and Conditioning.* Human Kinetics (Champaign, IL), 2000, page 269; *Medical Encyclopedia;* Losing Weight. A.D.A.M. Editorial. Medline, National Institutes of Health. January, 2004.

6. Walter C. Willet, M.D. *Eat, Drink, and Be Healthy.* Free Press (New York), 2003, pages 56–138.

7. Sharon Faelten, Ed. *Banish Your Belly, Butt & Thighs Forever!* Rodale, Inc. (Emmaus, PA), 2001, page 4.

CHAPTER 4

1. Wayne Westcott, Ph.D., CSCS, and Rita La Rosa Loud. *No More Cellulite.* Perigee (New York), 2003, pages 11–16.

2. Starbucks' Nutritional Information Comparison Table, www.starbucks.com, based on calories in 12-ounce latte with whole milk.

CHAPTER 5

All of the exercise guidelines were adapted from exercise guidelines designed by the American College of Sports Medicine and the National Strength and Conditioning Association. To read their guidelines, consult the following documents: Michael L. Pollock, Ph.D., et al. "The Recommended Quantity and Quality of Exercise for Developing and Maintaining Cardiorespiratory and Muscular Fitness, and Flexibility in Healthy Adults." *Medicine & Science in Sports & Exercise®*, vol. 30, no. 6, June 1998; the National Strength and Conditioning Association. *The NSCA Quick Series Guide to Basic Weight Training.* NSCA (Colorado Springs, CO), 1997.

1. Wayne Westcott, Ph.D. "Research on Advanced Strength Training." Naturalstrength.com, April 15, 2000.

2. Wayne Westcott, Ph.D. "Best of Both Worlds: Stretching and Strengthening." HealthWorld Online. www.healthy.net.

Chapter 6

1. Blandine Calais-Germain. *Anatomy of Movement.* Eastland Press (Seattle, WA), 1993, pages 40–43.

Chapter 7

1. Wayne Westcott, Ph.D. "Strength Training for Women." HealthWorld Online. www.healthy.net; Wayne Westcott, Ph.D., CSCS, and Rita La Rosa Loud. *No More Cellulite.* Perigee (New York), 2003, page 12.

NOTES

APPENDIX A

1. Adapted from information in *Sculpting Her Body Perfect*. Brad Schoenfeld. Human Kinetics (Champaign, IL), 2000.

Resources

While researching this book, I used a variety of fitness equipment, provided by the following companies:

RESISTANCE BANDS, TUBING, STABILITY BALLS AND AEROBICS STEPS

SPRI Products, Inc.
1600 Northwind Boulevard
Libertyville, IL 60048
800-222-7774
www.spriproducts.com

Sample products: aerobics steps; the UltraToner, the Xering, and Lex Loops rubber resistance tubing, the SPRI Xercise Ball stability ball

Sissel, Inc.
P.O. Box 729
Sumas, WA 98295
888-474-7735
www.sissel-online.com
Sample products: Ankle Tube and Fitband rubber resistance tubing, the Swiss Ball Pro stability ball

Stretchwell, Inc.
P.O. Box 3081
Warminster, PA 18974
888-369-2430
www.stretchwell.com
Sample products: Fit-Loops, Stretch-8, and Stretch-O rubber resistance tubing

Theraband
The Hygenic Corporation
Akron, OH 44310-2575

800-321-2135 (U.S.A. only); 330-633-8460 (Outside U.S.A.)
www.thera-band.com
Sample products: Theraband Resistive Exercise System bands
and tubing, SDS (Slow Deflate System) exercise and stability ball

STRENGTH TRAINING EQUIPMENT

TMG Fit
The McCorry Group, Inc.
105 Price Avenue
Berwyn, PA 19312
800-698-1498
www.tmgfit.com
Sample products: weighted vest, wrist and ankle weights

EDUCATION/INFORMATION

The American College of Sports Medicine (ACSM)
P.O. Box 1440
Indianapolis, IN 46202-1440
317-637-9200
www.acsm.org

RESOURCES

The American Council on Exercise (ACE)
4851 Paramount Drive
San Diego, CA 92123
800-825-3636, 858-279-8227
www.acefitness.org

The American Senior Fitness Association (SFA)
P.O. Box 2575
New Smyrna Beach, FL 32170
800-243-1478, 386-423-6634
www.seniorfitness.net

The National Strength and Conditioning Association (NSCA)
1885 Bob Johnson Drive
Colorado Springs, CO 80906
800-815-6826, 719-632-6722
www.nsca-lift.org

IDEA Health & Fitness Association (IDEA)
10455 Pacific Center Court
San Diego, CA 92121-4339
800-999-4332, 858-535-8979
www.ideafit.com

Resources

NUTRITION: SUGGESTED READING

Clark, Nancy, M.S., R.D. *Nancy Clark's Sports Nutrition Guidebook*. Human Kinetics (Champaign, IL), 2003.

Tribole, Evelyn, M.S., R.D. *Eating on the Run*. Human Kinetics (Champaign, IL), 2004.

Willet, Walter C., M.D. *Eat, Drink, and Be Healthy*. Free Press (New York), 2001.

STRETCHING: SUGGESTED READING

Blahnik, Jay. *Full-Body Flexibility*. Human Kinetics (Champaign, IL), 2004.

Westcott, Wayne, Ph.D. *Building Strength & Stamina*. Human Kinetics (Champaign, IL), 2003.

Index

INDEX

Index

INDEX

Index

INDEX

Index

INDEX

Index

INDEX